FACILITATED
STRETCHING

Robert E. McAtee
Pro-Active Massage Therapy
Colorado Springs, CO

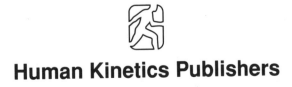

Human Kinetics Publishers

Library of Congress Cataloging-in-Publication Data

McAtee, Robert E. 1948-
    Facilitated stretching / Robert E.
McAtee.
      p. cm.
    Includes bibliographical references and index.
    ISBN 0-87322-420-5
    1. Stretching exercises. 2. Athletes. 3. Physical therapy.
    RA781.63.M33 1993
    613.7'11--dc20

92-36778
CIP

ISBN: 0-87322-420-5
    0-87322-867-7 (book and video VHS set)
    0-87322-868-5 (book and video PAL set)

Developmental Editor: Mary E. Fowler
Assistant Editors: Moyra Knight, Lisa Sotirelis
Copyeditor: Wendy Nelson
Proofreader: Pam Johnson
Indexer: Theresa J. Schaefer
Production Director: Ernie Noa
Typesetter: Kathleen Boudreau-Fuoss
Text Design and Interior Art: Keith Blomberg
Text Layout: Kathleen Boudreau-Fuoss
Cover Design: Jack Davis
Cover and Interior Photos: Wendy Pearce Nelson
Models: David L. Caldwell, Matt Carpenter, Jeff Charland, Pedro Cruz, Cliff Hong, Russia C. Madden, Jill
   Trenary, Dolly J. Wong, and Barry Helton
Printer: United Graphics

Human Kinetics books are available at special discounts for bulk purchase. Special editions or book excerpts can also be created to specification. For details, contact the Special Sales Manager at Human Kinetics.

Printed in the United States of America   10 9 8 7 6 5

Human Kinetics
P.O. Box 5076, Champaign, IL 61825-5076
1-800-747-4457

Canada: Human Kinetics, Box 24040, Windsor, ON N8Y 4Y9
1-800-465-7301 (in Canada only)

Europe: Human Kinetics, P.O. Box IW14, Leeds LS16 6TR, United Kingdom
(44) 1132 781708

Australia: Human Kinetics, 2 Ingrid Street, Clapham 5062, South Australia
(08) 371 3755

New Zealand: Human Kinetics, P.O. Box 105-231, Auckland 1
(09) 523 3462

To my wife, Trina, whose love and support have helped me "stretch" as a massage therapist, as a writer, and as a person

Contents

About the Authors   vii

Preface   ix

Acknowledgments   xi

Chapter 1   **Introduction to PNF Stretching**   **1**

The Development of PNF   1

The Neurophysiological Basis for PNF   3

Types of Stretching   5

Chapter 2   **Reviewing the Literature**   **9**

Current Research   10

Arguments Against PNF   10

Evidence Supporting PNF   11

Efficacy of PNF Today   12

Chapter 3   **Single-Muscle Stretches**   **13**

CRAC Technique   14

Stretches for the Lower Extremities   16

Stretches for the Upper Extremities   52

Stretches for the Torso   68

Chapter 4   **Using Spiral-Diagonal Patterns**   **77**

Applying Spiral-Diagonal Patterns to CRAC Stretching   78

Learning the Patterns   79

Stretches for the Upper Extremities   84
Stretches for the Lower Extremities   88

***Chapter 5*   Rehabilitation and PNF**   **93**
    Jeff Charland, RPT, ATC

Goals of Rehabilitation   94
The Many Uses for PNF   94
General Guidelines for Rehabilitation   94
Theoretical Case Study   95
A Typical PNF Rehabilitation Session   97

Glossary   101

References   103

Index   105

About the Authors

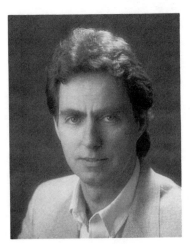

Robert McAtee

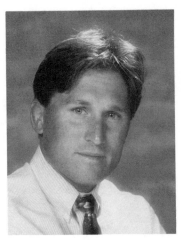

Jeff Charland, RPT, ATC

Robert McAtee has been a massage therapist since 1981, specializing in sport and orthopedic massage therapy. He has worked in both clinical settings and private practice and currently maintains a private sport massage practice in Colorado Springs, Colorado.

McAtee received his massage training at the Institute for Psycho-Structural Balancing in Los Angeles and San Diego and through the Sports Massage Training Institute (SMTI) in Costa Mesa, California. He has been designated a preferred therapist by SMTI and is a member of the National Sports Massage Team of the American Massage Therapy Association.

McAtee presents massage clinics to massage therapists, physical therapists, chiropractors, Olympic-caliber athletes and coaches, and amateur athletes. He is a former instructor at the Massage Training Institute in Encinitas, California, and teaches at the Colorado Springs Academy of Therapeutic Massage.

Jeff Charland is a 1983 graduate of the University of Wisconsin physical therapy program. His postgraduate study has focused on motor learning, biomechanics, and muscle energy technique.

Charland has worked extensively with college and Olympic-level athletes at the U.S. Olympic Training Center in Lake Placid, as an athletic trainer for Colorado College, and at the U.S. Olympic Festival (1991). He is the owner/director of Charland Physical Therapy Clinics of Colorado Springs, Colorado, which specialize in orthopedic and sport physical therapy.

Charland is a member of the American Physical Therapy Association and the National Athletic Trainers Association. He is also licensed as an emergency medical technician.

Preface

Proprioceptive neuromuscular facilitation (PNF) is a well-conceived, extremely effective physical therapy modality developed in the 1940s and 1950s to rehabilitate patients with paralysis. In the 1980s, sport therapists began using the stretching components of PNF with healthy athletes to increase their range of motion to improve performance and reduce the risk of injury.

Unfortunately, until now the material available on PNF has been highly technical and not suited for self-instruction. Most of it is written to physical therapists working with patients suffering from physical deficits. In *Facilitated Stretching* I provide selected PNF stretching techniques appropriate for healthy individuals and provide instructions with photos and illustrations to make your learning easy. This book is especially for sport massage therapists, athletic trainers, sport physicians, coaches, athletes, and anyone else who works with healthy, active people who wish to maintain or increase their range of motion.

I call the book *Facilitated Stretching* to clearly distinguish it from PNF techniques practiced as physical therapy. My goal is to demonstrate the valuable PNF stretching techniques available for use by and with healthy people.

The stretching techniques used in *Facilitated Stretching* are known as CRAC (contract-relax, antagonist-contract) stretches, and most of the major muscle groups are covered. Once you've learned the basic theory and technique, you can design stretches for almost any muscle or muscle group. I also have demonstrated the most common spiral-diagonal patterns used in PNF to promote flexibility and coordination throughout the entire range of motion of a leg or an arm. Whenever possible, I've included instructions for self-stretching, so the participant can be fully involved in maintaining newly achieved range of motion.

The facilitated stretching techniques presented here are not meant to replace the daily stretching program that every sportsperson already should have in place. PNF is used to make quick gains in range of motion, and a daily static stretching program is important to maintain those gains.

Range of motion is critical to athletic performance—lack of it contributes to improper biomechanics, fatigue, and overuse injuries. If you want to help athletes and active adults achieve their optimum range of motion for improved performance, this book is for you.

Acknowledgments

Although the process of writing is a solitary one (especially during the late-night sessions when the rest of the household is in dreamland), the production of a book like this is the result of support and contributions from many people. For my book, the many people include these:

John Harris, friend and teacher, first introduced me to PNF and its usefulness in working with athletes. He later provided the opportunity, through the Massage Training Institute, for me to really learn PNF stretching by teaching it to others. John also inspired me to begin writing about sport massage and originated the project that has evolved into this book.

Karen Thompson, RPT, another good friend, simplified some of the more complex areas of PNF for me so that I could explain them more clearly in these pages. She also reviewed the early drafts of the manuscript and made helpful suggestions for improvement.

Jeff Charland, RPT, AT, C, started out as a reviewer of the early draft of the book and ended up agreeing to write chapter 5. His comments and suggestions have been thoughtful, timely, and extremely beneficial.

Ron Fisher, RPT, generously shared his knowledge and his third edition of Voss et al.

Tim Bonack, RPT, who never loans his books, graciously made an exception and allowed me the extended use of his second edition of Voss et al., which he had providentially highlighted during his student days.

Ed Burke generously reviewed my preliminary proposal, gave constructive criticism, and guided me to Human Kinetics Publishers.

Mary Fowler, my developmental editor, was always available to answer my questions. Her skill in clarifying and organizing the material has significantly improved the final form of the book.

Rainer Martens, publisher, saw the potential for this book and took a chance on an unproven writer.

1

Introduction to PNF Stretching

Most of us know that stretching is an important part of training for any sport and that there are many ways to stretch. Over the past 10 years, PNF (proprioceptive neuromuscular facilitation) has gained popularity. PNF is a form of stretching that uses an isometric contraction prior to the stretch to achieve greater gains than from stretching alone.

Dramatic gains in flexibility are possible in a very short time with this technique, due to the creative use of a few neurological mechanisms to optimize a muscle's ability to lengthen. In this chapter, you'll learn the basics of PNF theory; in chapter 3 you will learn how to actually do the stretching. A thorough grounding in the *why* of PNF will make the *how* easier in daily practice. Our objectives in this chapter are to

- provide brief account of how PNF evolved,
- explain the neurophysiological basis for PNF as theorized by the founders of this technique, and
- consider where PNF fits in with the other types of stretching methods.

The Development of PNF

Proprioceptive neuromuscular facilitation is a treatment modality developed in the late 1940s and early 1950s by Herman Kabat, MD, PhD, with the primary assistance of two physical therapists, Margaret "Maggie" Knott and Dorothy Voss. Dr. Kabat was a neurophysiologist who believed that the principles of neurophysiological development should be applied in the rehabilitation of polio patients with paralysis. Prior to the development of PNF techniques, paralyzed patients had been rehabilitated using a method that emphasized "one motion, one joint, one muscle at a time" (Voss, Ionta, & Myers, 1985). With backing from Henry Kaiser, the industrialist, Dr. Kabat founded the Kabat-Kaiser Institute (KKI) in Washington, DC, in 1946 and began working with patients to find combinations and patterns of movement that were consistent with neurophysiological theory.

Spiral-Diagonal Patterns

Dr. Kabat's experimentation led him to realize that movement occurs in spiral-diagonal patterns. The motions required when you comb your hair, swing a golf club, or kick a ball all have spiral and diagonal components; that is, they occur in three planes of motion. If you look at Figure 1.1, you can see that the bowler's arms are moving through three planes: front to back, down to up, and right to left. You'll also notice the spiral component of his motion if you look at the rotation of his arms. Even when you walk, your arms move back and forth, up and down, and slightly across the front of your body: three planes.

Kabat and Maggie Knott believed that using natural patterns of movement would stimulate the nervous system more normally than would therapy that isolated each muscle. Kabat combined these patterns with techniques to develop strength and flexibility based on the principles of successive induction, reciprocal innervation, and irradiation developed by neurophysiologist Charles Sherrington, which are discussed in a later section.

PNF in the 1950s

By 1951, Kabat and Knott had identified and were using nine techniques for rehabilitating muscles. By this time there were two more Kabat-Kaiser Institutes, both in California (in Vallejo and Santa Monica). Dorothy Voss became interested in PNF in 1950 and spent 6

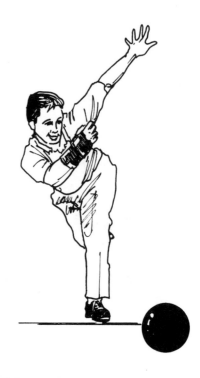

Figure 1.1   The bowler illustrates arm movement traveling through three planes of motion: front to back, down to up, right to left.

weeks at KKI Vallejo in 1951 learning from and working with Maggie Knott. She subsequently was hired as Knott's assistant at Vallejo in 1952. She and Knott realized that PNF was more than a system for the treatment of paralysis; it was a new way of thinking about and using movement and therapeutic exercise. In 1952 Knott and Voss began presenting workshops to train other physical therapists in the PNF methods. By 1954, they were conducting 2-week trainings, first at KKI Vallejo, then at Boston University. During the 1960s, PNF courses became available through physical therapy departments at several universities, and its popularity continued to grow.

PNF in the Present

By the late 1970s, physical therapists and athletic trainers had begun using PNF techniques to facilitate flexibility and range of motion in healthy people. Practitioners began experimenting with variations of the standard techniques, adapting them to their own needs. Some of the terminology changed, and versions of PNF stretching became known as Scientific Stretching for Sport (3-S technique), NF technique, and modified PNF. As word of the effectiveness of PNF stretching spread, other sport practitioners, including massage therapists, sport physical therapists, athletic trainers, coaches, and sport physicians, began using these techniques.

PNF in the Future

The rapid growth in sports medicine in the 1980s has fueled the search by practitioners for effective, efficient techniques for improving sport performance. The adaptation of PNF stretching techniques for use with athletes opened the door for its current popularity among sport health practitioners. The use of PNF will continue to expand as therapists and athletes realize the gains in flexibility it makes possible.

The Neurophysiological Basis for PNF

PNF is based on several neurophysiological mechanisms. Understanding these various muscle contractions and reflexes provides you with necessary insight into the basis of PNF practices and helps prevent misuse of the procedures.

Types of Muscle Contractions

Two types of muscle contractions, isotonic and isometric, are used in applying the principles of PNF. You need to clearly understand their differences to properly perform PNF stretching.

Isotonic

An isotonic muscle contraction is a voluntary contraction that causes movement. There are two types of isotonic contractions: concentric, in which the muscle shortens as it works, and eccentric, in which the muscle exerts force while being lengthened by an outside force. A concentric isotonic contraction of the pectoral muscles, for example, occurs when you bring your hands into the prayer position (Figure 1.2). An eccentric contraction of the pectorals occurs if someone else pulls your hands apart while you resist.

Isometric

An isometric muscle contraction is a voluntary concentric contraction in which no joint movement occurs and muscle length is unchanged. If you place your hands in the prayer position, then push, the push isometrically contracts the pectoral muscles.

Stretch Reflexes

Reflexes are automatic responses designed to protect the body. Stretch reflexes protect the muscles and joints from injury due to overstretching or excessive strain.

Myotatic Stretch Reflex

The myotatic stretch reflex prevents a muscle from stretching too far too fast, which protects the joint from injury. The stretch reflex is mediated through the muscle spindle cells (Figure 1.3). Located in the muscle belly, the spindle

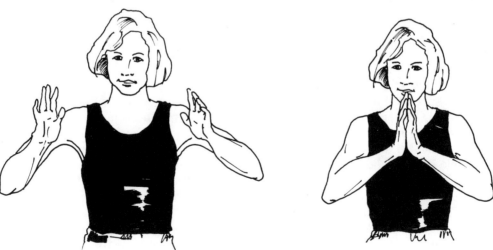

Figure 1.2 A concentric isotonic contraction of the pectoral muscles.

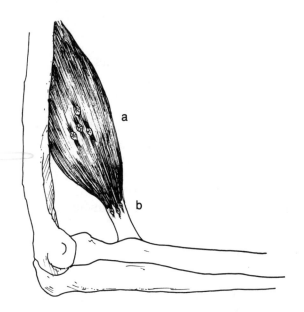

Figure 1.3 (a) Muscle spindle cells and (b) Golgi tendon organs.

cells monitor the tonus of the muscle. They sense changes in muscle length and the speed of those changes. When a muscle lengthens too quickly, the spindle cell is stimulated and reflexively causes the muscle to contract, resisting the lengthening and thereby preventing overstretching of the joint.

Inverse Stretch Reflex

The inverse stretch reflex (also called autogenic inhibition) is the firing of the Golgi tendon organs (GTOs) to inhibit, or relax, a muscle. The Golgi organs are located in the muscle tendon and monitor the amount of strain on the tendon (Figure 1.3). Strain develops in the tendon when the muscle contracts and pulls on it. Theoretically, when a maximal contraction is elicited from a muscle, the inverse stretch reflex, mediated by the GTOs, should cause it to relax. This is the basis for the theory of postisometric relaxation, which postulates that a muscle is neurologically relaxed, and therefore more easily stretched, following a maximal isometric contraction. Strain is also sensed by the GTOs when the muscle is stretched, because the tendon is once again being pulled. When a muscle stretch is held, the pull on the tendons should stimulate the GTOs and cause the muscle to relax and lengthen further to reduce the chances of muscle tearing.

It's easy to get confused about the functions of spindle cells and GTOs. Just remember that the spindle cells reflexively cause the muscle to contract, and the GTOs reflexively cause the muscle to relax. Both reflexes are protective.

Sherrington's Laws

Kabat based much of the theoretical structure of PNF on the work of Charles Sherrington, whose research in the early to mid-1900s helped develop a model for how the neuromuscular system operates. Kabat incorporated Sherrington's laws of successive induction, reciprocal innervation, and irradiation into his work on PNF. If you understand these principles, you will find it easier to learn the PNF stretching technique.

Successive Induction

Successive induction is the isometric or isotonic contraction of one muscle, followed immediately by the contraction of its antagonist (the opposing muscle). Sherrington believed that flexion enhances extension and that extension enhances flexion. The same applies to adduction and abduction. In some PNF techniques, successive induction is repeated several times to promote strength and flexibility.

Reciprocal Innervation

Reciprocal innervation (or reciprocal inhibition) is a reflex loop mediated by the muscle spindle cell. It causes one muscle to relax (be inhibited from contracting) when the opposing muscle (the antagonist) contracts. This allows movement to occur around a joint. For instance, when the quadriceps muscle contracts, the hamstring is reciprocally inhibited, thereby allowing the knee to straighten (Figure 1.4).

Irradiation

Irradiation occurs when a maximal contraction of the muscle is achieved by applying resistance. The excitation of the primary muscle flows out (irradiates) to synergistic muscles, which then become involved to overcome the resistance. Also known as recruitment, this can be seen in any weight room. When a person tries to lift a heavy weight, the body automatically recruits additional muscles to spread the work and keep the primary muscle from being overpowered (Figure 1.5, a and b).

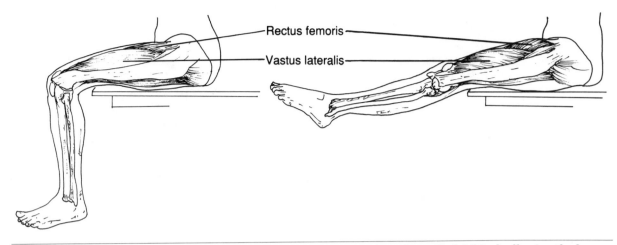

Figure 1.4   When the quadriceps muscle contracts, the hamstring is reciprocally inhibited, allowing the knee to straighten.

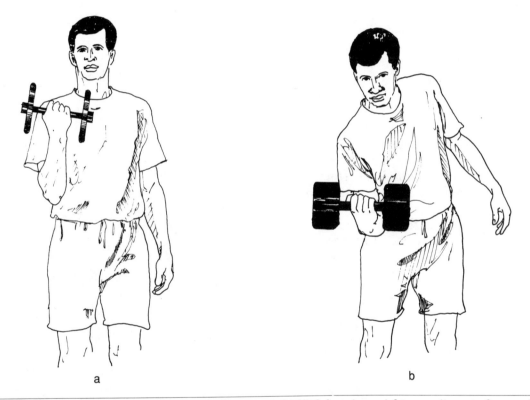

a   b

Figure 1.5   (a) Proper form during a low-weight bicep curl. (b) With heavier weight, recruitment of synergistic muscles is likely, causing shoulder elevation and side-bending.

Types of Stretching

There are several types of stretching in use for sport. Knowing their differences and similarities will help you understand the research presented in chapter 2 and see why PNF stretching is a valuable addition to your stretching repertoire.

Static Stretching

Static stretching has been popularized by Bob Anderson's book *Stretching* (1984). The muscle to be stretched (the target muscle) is lengthened slowly (to inhibit the firing of the stretch reflex) and held in a comfortable range for 15 to 30 s. As the position is held, the feeling of

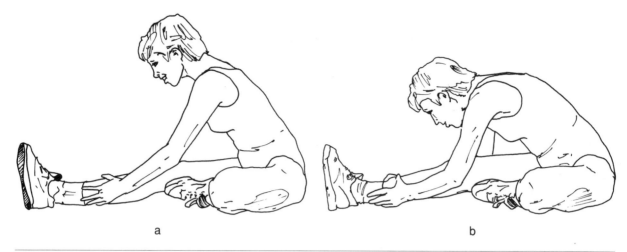

Figure 1.6   One example of a static stretch is the seated hamstring stretch. The stretch (a) begins and (b) deepens after 15 to 30 s.

stretch diminishes (theoretically, due to the inverse stretch reflex), and the stretcher moves gently into a deeper stretch and holds again (Figure 1.6, a and b).

Ballistic Stretching

Ballistic, or dynamic, stretching is done using rapid bouncing movements, to force the target muscle to elongate (Figure 1.7). This type of stretching may evoke a strong stretch reflex and leave the muscle shorter than its prestretching length. Beaulieu (1981) asserts that ballistic stretching creates more than twice the tension in the target muscle, compared to a static stretch. This increases the likelihood of tearing the muscle, because the

rapid bouncing does not allow enough time for the inverse stretch reflex to be engaged and relax the muscle.

Passive Stretching

Passive stretching is done to the stretcher by a partner or coach; it can be ballistic or static. The stretcher relaxes, and the partner moves the limb being stretched to gain new range of motion (Figure 1.8). Passive stretching is of-

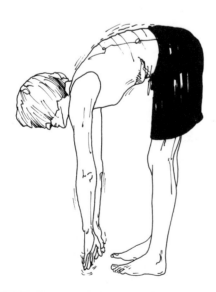

Figure 1.7   Ballistic stretching is done using rapid, bouncing movements.

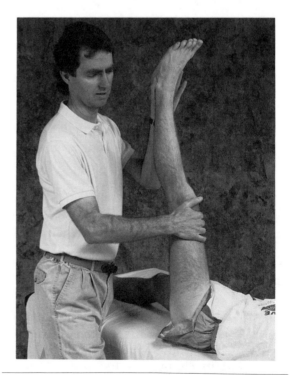

Figure 1.8   Passive stretching is done to the stretcher by a partner.

ten used to increase flexibility at the extremes of range of motion, as in gymnastics, where maximum flexibility is crucial for performance. Done carelessly or with poor form, passive stretching can cause muscle injury. It is risky because the person assisting the stretching cannot feel the sensations of the stretcher and may overstretch the muscle.

PNF Stretching

PNF stretching is one component of the entire PNF repertoire. Versions of PNF stretching are referred to as modified PNF (Moore & Hutton, 1980; Cornelius & Craft-Hamm, 1988), NF (Surburg, 1981) and Scientific Stretching for Sport (3-S technique; Holt, 1976). The following PNF patterns are commonly used to increase flexibility.

Hold-Relax

Hold-relax (HR) is generally used if range of motion is extremely limited or if active move-

ment causes pain. The stretcher holds the limb at its lengthened range of motion and isometrically resists the therapist's attempt to move the limb into a deeper stretch. The stretcher then relaxes, and the limb is moved passively into the new range (Figure 1.9, a and b). Kabat theorized that the strong isometric contraction would recruit more muscle fibers (irradiation) and then fire the inverse stretch reflex, relaxing the target muscle and permitting further stretch.

Contract-Relax

Contract-relax (CR) is similar to hold-relax. The difference is that the therapist provides resistance as the stretcher isometrically attempts to move the limb into the shortened range of the target muscle. The stretcher then relaxes, and the limb is moved passively into the new range. CR is preferable to HR when range of motion is good and when motion is pain-free.

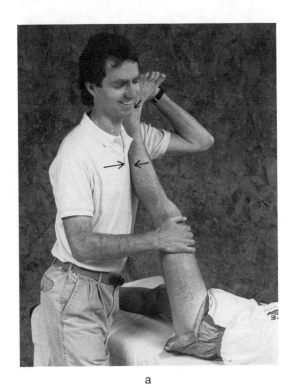

a

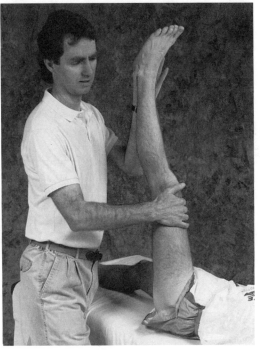

b

Figure 1.9   (a) The PNF hold-relax hamstring stretch. The arrows indicate the stretcher's isometric contraction and the partner's force to overcome it. (b) The stretcher is passively moved into a deeper stretch.

CRAC

Contract-relax, antagonist-contract (CRAC) is performed much the same as CR, except that after the isometric contraction, the stretcher actively moves the limb into the new range of motion (Figure 1.10, a and b). This active contraction of the antagonist is thought to elicit reciprocal inhibition of the target muscle, thereby allowing a deeper stretch.

Now that you have a feel for how PNF developed and understand its basic terminology, we can review the current research concerning the various aspects of PNF stretching.

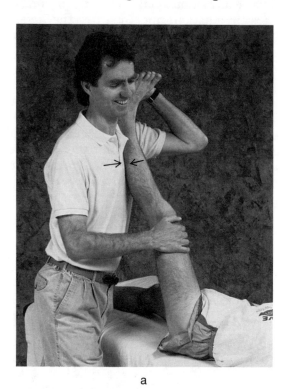

a

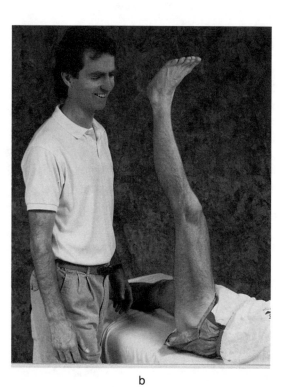

b

Figure 1.10 (a) The CRAC hamstring stretch. The arrows indicate the partner's resistance as the stretcher increases the force of his isometric contraction. (b) The stretcher actively moves into a deeper stretch with no help from his partner. Here, the partner has removed his hands from the stretcher to demonstrate the stretcher's active movement. In an actual stretch, the partner maintains the stretcher's knee extension.

2

Reviewing the Literature

PNF was developed through trial and error, in a clinical setting, based on hypotheses formed by Dr. Kabat from his synthesis of "the work of [Arnold] Gesell and [George] Coghill on motor development, the findings of [Charles] Sherrington and [Ivan] Pavlov on habit action and reflexes, and the work of [Ernst] Gellhorn on proprioception and cortically controlled movement" (Surburg, 1981, pp. 115-116). The technique evolved to include only the patterns of movement that worked most effectively with patients. Those patterns, by no coincidence, are similar to the functional patterns that occur naturally in daily activities. It was only after PNF was in wide use that controlled studies were undertaken to examine its effectiveness and to see if the neurophysiological principles on which it is based could be validated.

In this chapter, we will

- examine the current research on the effectiveness of PNF for stretching,
- review studies related to the neurophysiological basis of PNF, and
- consider the efficacy of PNF stretching for sport today.

Current Research

Researchers have begun to study PNF stretching in detail to see whether it is more effective than other types of stretching and, if so, whether this is due to the neurological mechanisms proposed by Kabat.

As is common in research, many of these studies raise more questions than they answer. This is good, because controversy and unanswered questions stimulate thought, discussion, and further investigation of the mechanisms at work.

Arguments Against PNF

A number of studies have investigated whether PNF stretching is more effective than other types. None of the studies I reviewed found PNF to be less effective, but several researchers recommend other types of stretching over PNF for two reasons:

- PNF is no more effective than other forms of stretching and is too complex.
- There are risks of injury that other forms of stretching eliminate.

The Complexities of PNF

The following studies have concluded that, although PNF works, it is no more effective than other types of stretching. Many of these authors believe that, because PNF is more complicated to use, it's better to use the more conventional forms of stretching.

Medeiros, Smidt, Burmeister, and Soderberg (1977) compared the effects of passive stretching with isometric contractions on range of motion at the hip joint. Testing indicated that both groups significantly increased hip flexion compared to the control group, but there was no significant difference in the gains made by the isometric group compared to the passive stretch group.

Lucas and Koslow (1984) compared static, dynamic, and PNF stretching. They found that all three were effective in increasing the flexibility of the hamstring and gastrocnemius muscles and that no method produced significantly superior results. They also noted that total stretching time may influence effectiveness. They refer to two studies with short treat-

ment times (18 and 12 min) that found PNF to be better, compared to their own study, and one other with longer treatment times (105 and 90 min) that found no significant differences between the three types of stretching.

Condon and Hutton (1987) compared static stretching and three PNF techniques for increasing dorsiflexion of the ankle and concluded that there was no significant difference between techniques.

Potential Risks

Several authors have discussed possible risks inherent in using PNF techniques. Their concerns are valid and must be considered if we are to avoid injury when using PNF stretching.

Increased EMG Activity

Beaulieu (1981) points out that the isometric contraction preceding a PNF stretch has been shown by Moore and Hutton (1980) to promote higher electromyographic (EMG) readings in the target muscle and, theoretically, puts the muscle at higher risk of injury during the stretch phase. (Electromyography is a way of measuring the electrical activity of a muscle. A relaxed muscle is quieter electrically than an active one.)

Investigators in two other EMG studies (Condon & Hutton, 1987; Osternig, Robertson, Troxel, & Hansen, 1987) also noted higher EMG readings in the target muscle during the antagonist contraction that lengthens the target muscle. These findings seem to indicate that the target muscle is less relaxed following an isometric contraction, or that reciprocal inhibition is not occurring as the antagonist contracts, or both. Accordingly, these authors all recommend static stretching as being safer than PNF.

Inattentive Partners

Surburg (1983) discusses the potential injury risks associated with partner (passive) stretching. He believes that lack of attention, improper training, and faulty performance of the techniques contribute to the risk of injury in partner stretching. He correctly points out that these considerations apply to any stretching technique.

Cardiovascular Complications

Cornelius (1983) mentions the potential risk of increased systolic blood pressure as a result of the Valsalva maneuver during the isometric contraction phase of PNF and the implications for those with hypertension. (The Valsalva maneuver occurs when you try to exhale against a closed glottis, as often happens when performing an isometric contraction or lifting a heavy weight. This sets up a series of reactions that can lead to a momentary increase in blood pressure.) However, in a later study (Cornelius & Craft-Hamm, 1988) he determined that increases in blood pressure were not significant compared to baseline measures and that the short duration of PNF techniques produced no risks for people who have hypertension without other symptoms.

Neurological Studies

Research has also been done to determine if the neurological mechanisms thought to be responsible for the effectiveness of PNF techniques are, in fact, responsible. The studies I reviewed throw into question the basic assumptions upon which PNF techniques are based.

Sapega, Quedenfeld, Moyer, and Butler (1981) reviewed relevant research on the factors that contribute to range of motion. They state that "the weight of laboratory evidence indicates that when a relaxed muscle is physically stretched, most, if not all, of the resistance to stretch is derived from the extensive connective tissue framework and sheathing within and around the muscle, *not from the myofibrillar elements*" (p. 58, emphasis added).

Taylor, Dalton, Seaber, and Garrett (1990) conducted a creative study of the viscoelastic properties of muscle-tendon units and how they are affected by stretching. These authors believe that the viscoelastic properties of the muscle-tendon unit are responsible for the gains made through stretching. Their results indicate that reflex activity has no influence on the results of several stretching procedures.

A series of studies by various researchers using electromyography found levels of electrical activity in the target muscle that indicate the absence of reciprocal or autogenic inhibition during PNF procedures (Moore & Hutton, 1980; Cornelius, 1983; Condon & Hutton, 1987; Osternig et al., 1987, 1990).

These neurological studies raise serious questions about the validity of Kabat's and others' hypotheses concerning mechanisms like the stretch reflex, reciprocal innervation, and autogenic inhibition and their contribution to the effectiveness of PNF techniques.

Evidence Supporting PNF

Eight of the 14 studies I reviewed (57%) found that PNF is significantly more effective for increasing range of motion and flexibility than either static, ballistic, or passive stretching.

Tanigawa (1972) compared passive stretching with PNF for the hamstring. He determined that PNF increased passive hip flexion faster, and to a greater extent, than did passive stretching.

Moore and Hutton (1980) used electromyography to investigate the differences between static stretching and two PNF techniques. Although their findings raised questions about the value of using isometric contraction before a stretch, their results indicated that CRAC stretches were more effective than static stretching for improving flexibility.

Sady, Wortman, and Blanke (1982) compared the effects of ballistic, static, and PNF stretching on shoulder, trunk, and hamstring flexibility. They found that only the PNF technique (CRAC) significantly increased range of motion compared to the control group. These researchers also noted that individual flexibility changed from day to day, compared to the baseline flexibility established for each subject in the study. In addition, they found flexibility to be highly variable within the body; their subjects increased flexibility in the hamstrings to a greater extent than in the trunk muscles. They theorized that this may be due to daily postural mechanics that demand more flexibility of the trunk muscles than the hamstrings. Therefore, the hamstrings have a greater range of possible improvement.

Prentice (1983) compared static stretching and PNF for increasing flexibility at the hip joint and found that, although both methods were effective, PNF was significantly better than static stretching. Cornelius and Craft-Hamm (1988) compared passive stretching and three types of PNF while investigating their effects on arterial blood pressure. They determined that the PNF techniques were more effective than passive stretching. They also found that there were no significant increases in arterial blood pressure during PNF and concluded that the benefits of PNF outweigh any potential risk of elevated blood pressure.

Etnyre and Abraham (1986) compared static stretching to PNF (CR and CRAC) for increasing range of motion at the ankle joint. They determined that CRAC is more effective than CR, which is more effective than static stretching, for improving dorsiflexion at the ankle. In two similar EMG studies, Osternig et al. (1987, 1990) concluded that PNF is more effective than static stretching, although PNF evokes higher EMG activity in the target muscle.

Efficacy of PNF Today

If all these conflicting reports are confusing, don't worry. It's common in research of this type that some studies are positive and others negative. Even though we may not fully understand how or why PNF techniques work, it is clear that, at the minimum, PNF is as effective as other types of stretching. We also need to recognize that research often lags behind practical experience. Many therapists who use PNF believe strongly, based on their clinical experience, that PNF is superior, because it's a form of stretching that more closely approximates "natural" movement.

Your efforts to learn and use this method will be rewarded by greater gains in range of motion and flexibility. As more studies are conducted, a clearer picture will emerge to help us understand just what mechanisms are at work in PNF. This clearer understanding will enable us to use PNF stretching even more effectively in the future.

3

Single-Muscle Stretches

PNF techniques were developed as patterns of movement to increase strength, coordination, and flexibility through entire ranges of motion. Sometimes, with healthy people, we want to focus on just one muscle. This chapter presents PNF stretches that you can use to stretch one muscle at a time. These single-muscle stretches are valuable for developing flexibility in a specific muscle or muscle group and are simpler than the spiral-diagonal patterns covered in chapter 4, because they are performed in a single plane of motion. You can also use these stretches for softening hypertonic (too-tight) muscles to reduce the discomfort of deep massage or trigger-point work.

The PNF stretches presented here are not meant to replace the daily stretching program that every athlete should already have in place. PNF is used to make quick gains in range of motion and flexibility, and daily static stretching is important to maintain those gains.

Our objectives in this chapter are to

- define the PNF technique we're using,
- outline the steps used in performing a single-muscle PNF stretch, and
- provide detailed instructions and ample illustrations to demonstrate, one by one, stretches for the muscles of the leg, arm, and torso.

CRAC Technique

We will be using the CRAC (contract-relax, antagonist-contract) stretching technique exclusively. CRAC is a modified form of PNF in which the stretcher performs all of the stretching, and you act only as the facilitator. For example, during the hamstring stretch, the stretcher begins by actively moving the leg to the starting position, then isometrically contracts, then relaxes, the hamstring, as you provide resistance. The stretcher then actively raises the leg higher by contracting the antagonists (in this case, the quadriceps and psoas) to deepen the stretch.

In the available research that included CRAC techniques, CRAC was found to be the most effective in achieving gains in range of motion (Moore & Hutton, 1980; Cornelius, 1983; Etnyre & Abraham, 1986). CRAC stretches are also the safest PNF stretches, because there is no passive movement involved—the stretcher performs all of the stretching. You act only as a facilitator for the technique and make no attempt to increase the stretch. This factor addresses the concern of some investigators (Beaulieu, 1981; Surburg, 1983) that poorly trained or inattentive partners could cause injury by being too vigorous in moving the limb to a new range of motion.

The following sections explain and illustrate the most useful PNF stretches, done either with a partner or as self-stretches. Once you understand the basics of the CRAC technique, you can use it with almost any muscle or muscle group.

Using Less-Than-Maximal Contractions

When I was teaching at the Massage Training Institute, we began using less-than-maximal isometric contractions during PNF stretching as a safety measure. This prevented injury to our students as they were learning these techniques. Imagine how easy it would be for a 6-ft-2-in., 180-lb stretcher to overpower a 5-ft-6-in., 115-lb partner during a PNF stretching routine if the stretcher were using all his or her strength. We discovered that by using less-than-maximal contractions the stretcher experienced less discomfort during the stretch and still made excellent gains in flexibility. It is also much less tiring for the partner. Therefore, the instruc-tions for each stretch ask for a less-than-maximal isometric contraction.

CRAC Stretching Procedures

PNF stretching is best done with a partner, although many of the stretches can be done alone. Self-stretching is demonstrated in the text when it is applicable. These are the steps in a partner-assisted PNF stretch:

1. Actively lengthen the muscle to be stretched (the target muscle) to its maximal pain-free end of range. For example, if you wish to stretch the hamstring, have the stretcher lie on his back and contract his quadriceps and psoas (hip flexors) to actively lift the leg as high as possible, keeping the knee straight. This stretches the hamstring to its end of range.

2. Position yourself to serve as resistance (an "immovable object") for the stretcher to isometrically contract the target muscle against (Figure 3.1).

3. The stretcher then isometrically contracts the target muscle (hamstring) against your resistance. (Remember, an isometric con-

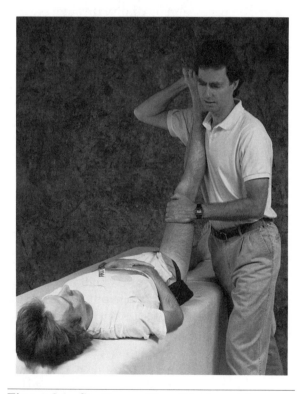

Figure 3.1   Starting position of the hamstring stretch (right leg). Support the stretcher's leg using proper biomechanics.

traction is one in which no movement occurs.) The contraction should begin gradually and build to 50% to 100% of maximum in a controlled manner. Muscles need oxygen to work properly, so the stretcher (and you) should be sure to continue breathing during the stretch. The isometric contraction is held for approximately 6 s.

4. The stretcher then relaxes and breathes deeply. This deep breath allows the nervous system to prepare for the next step; too rapid a change of direction may cause the muscle to tear. Maintain the limb in the starting position while the stretcher relaxes.

5. The stretcher now contracts the antagonist (the opposing muscle—in this case the quads and psoas) and pulls the target muscle into a deeper stretch. *Do not push to deepen the stretch* (Figure 3.2).

6. You now move into the new position to once again offer resistance.

7. Repeat the process 3 to 5 times.

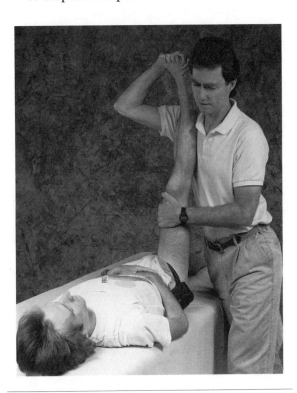

Figure 3.2 The stretcher actively deepens the stretch.

Stretching should be pain-free. If the stretcher experiences pain, try repositioning the limb, or use less force during the isometric contraction. If pain persists, don't use PNF until you know the cause of the pain.

Stretch Moderately

If the muscles being stretched are deconditioned, the stretcher may experience muscle fatigue and delayed-onset soreness the day after performing CRAC stretches. To avoid these effects with deconditioned muscles, never elicit more than 50% of muscular strength in the isometric phase of the stretch, and never repeat more than twice. Accept small gains with each stretch.

Well-conditioned athletes can often exert up to 100% of their strength with no problem, but I still recommend using less than full force. The gains achieved will be similar, and moderate gains are preferable to dramatic changes in muscle length. Too great an increase in flexibility in too short a time puts excessive demands on antagonist muscles to contract to new, shorter positions, which can lead to spasm or the firing of trigger points. For example, when the quadriceps group is lengthened through PNF, the hamstrings are able to contract more fully, often to a position they could not achieve before. This contraction may induce spasm. It is better to gain flexibility in the quads more slowly, to give the hamstrings time to adapt.

Use Good Biomechanics

Your body mechanics are extremely important during all phases of stretching, most especially during the isometric phase. If you are inattentive to your posture, you place yourself at risk for excessive fatigue and possible injury as you resist the stretcher's strong isometric contractions.

STRETCHES FOR THE LOWER EXTREMITIES

Flexibility in the hips and legs is important to success in most sports. When a muscle is chronically shortened, it cannot develop its full power when called upon to contract. At the same time, a chronically short muscle will limit range of motion. For instance, a runner with tight hamstrings will have a limited stride length and have to take more steps over a given distance than would be required with more flexibility. These stretches will help to develop flexibility in the major muscles of the hips and legs, which will contribute to improved athletic performance.

Each of the following sections covers one muscle or muscle group. The format is designed to provide you with the information you need to use PNF most effectively. Please be sure to read the special notes and cautions before doing any stretching. Each section is presented as follows:

- Origin, insertion, and action of muscle(s), with illustration
- Functional assessment for normal range of motion
- Special notes and cautions
- Detailed stretching instructions, with illustrations
- Self-stretching instructions, where appropriate, with illustrations
- Alternative stretching instructions, where appropriate, with illustrations

HAMSTRINGS

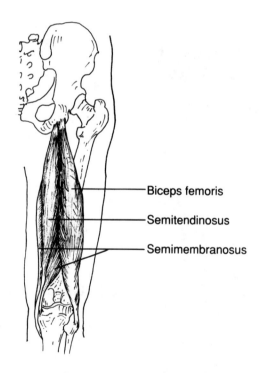

Biceps Femoris

Origin	Insertion	Action
Long head: ischial tuberosity	Head of fibula	Long head: extension of hip
Short head: linea aspera of femur		Both heads: knee flexion, lateral rotation of the leg with the knee flexed

Semimembranosus, Semitendinosus

Origin	Insertion	Action
Ischial tuberosity	SM: posteromedial tibial condyle ST: anterior proximal tibial shaft (pes anserine)	Hip extension, knee flexion, medial rotation of the leg with the knee flexed

Functional Assessment

Check range of motion (Figure 3.3). Hip flexion to 90° with the leg straight is optimal. Any less may shorten the athlete's stride in running. If less than 90°, do PNF stretching.

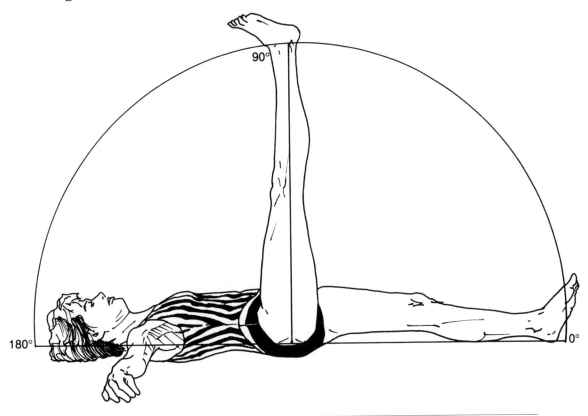

Figure 3.3   Hip flexion to 90° with the knee straight is ideal.

Instruction

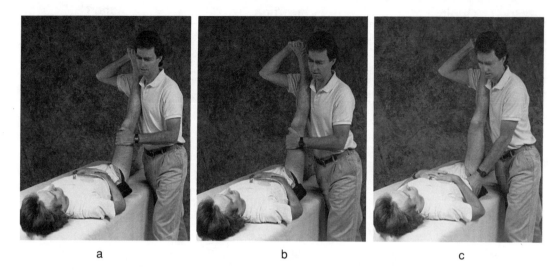

a   b   c

Figure 3.4   (a) Starting position of the hamstring stretch (right leg). (b) The stretcher actively deepens the stretch. (c) Stabilize the hip with your hand.

1. The stretcher is supine.

2. The stretcher lifts his leg, with the knee straight, as high as possible. This lengthens the hamstring to its pain-free end of range.

3. Offer resistance to the isometric contraction of the hamstring (no movement), at the same time making sure that the stretcher keeps his hips on the table (Figure 3.4a).

4. The stretcher pushes his heel toward the table, isometrically contracting the hamstring, for 6 s. The stretcher begins slowly and builds to 50% to 100% of maximum contraction, breathing throughout.

5. The stretcher relaxes, breathes deeply, then contracts his hip flexors (quads and psoas) to lift the leg higher, with the knee straight (Figure 3.4b). This deepens the hamstring stretch. *Never push to deepen the stretch*. As the stretcher lifts his leg higher, hold the knee straight and move in to offer resistance again.

6. Repeat 3 to 5 times.

7. The stretcher must keep his hips flat on the table. If necessary, stabilize them with your hand (Figure 3.4c).

Stretching should be pain-free. If the stretcher experiences pain, reposition the leg, or use less force during the isometric contraction. If pain persists, don't use PNF until you know the cause of the pain.

Self-Stretching

The stretcher's procedure differs from the preceding steps as follows:

- The stretcher uses a towel wrapped around the heel to provide resistance to the hamstring contraction. The towel replaces the partner. The stretcher should never pull on the towel to deepen the stretch (Figure 3.5).
- Figure 3.6 illustrates another option for self-stretching. The stretcher lies in a doorway and uses the doorjamb to provide resistance to the hamstring contraction, then moves forward following each round of stretching.

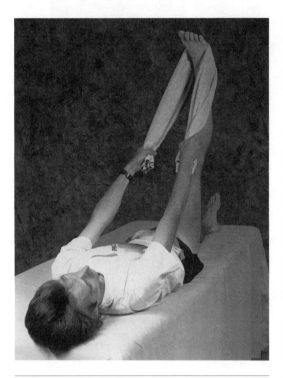
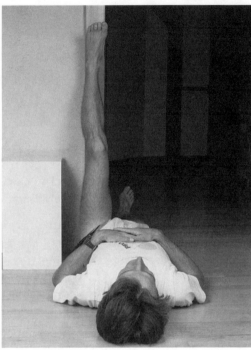

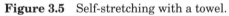

Figure 3.5 Self-stretching with a towel.   **Figure 3.6** Self-stretching in a doorway.

Alternative Instruction

This is a better stretch for people with very short hamstrings. Once they've achieved more flexibility, you can begin to use the standard positioning.

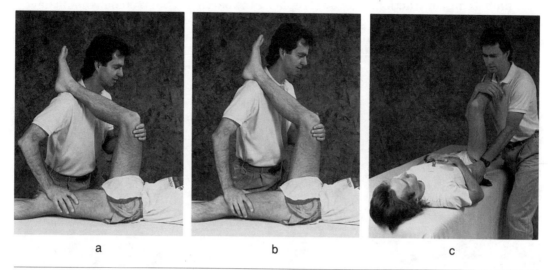

Figure 3.7   Alternate hamstring stretch: (a) Initiation with the right knee bent. Support the stretcher's leg. (b) The stretcher actively deepens the stretch. (c) Stabilize the stretcher's hip.

1. The stretcher lies supine and lifts his leg, with the knee bent, as high as possible. This lengthens the hamstring to its pain-free end of range.

2. Offer resistance to the isometric contraction of the hamstring (Figure 3.7a).

3. The stretcher pushes his heel toward the table, isometrically contracting the hamstring, for 6 s. The stretcher begins slowly and builds to 50% to 100% of maximum contraction, breathing throughout.

4. The stretcher relaxes, breathes deeply, then contracts his quadriceps to straighten the knee (Figure 3.7b). This deepens the hamstring stretch. *Never push to deepen the stretch*.

5. Repeat 3 to 5 times.

6. The stretcher must keep his hips flat on the table, especially during the isometric phase. If necessary, stabilize them with your hand (Figure 3.7c).

Stretching should be pain-free. If the stretcher experiences pain, reposition the leg, or use less force during the isometric contraction. If pain persists, don't use PNF until you know the cause of the pain.

QUADRICEPS

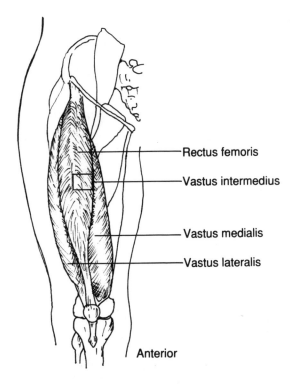

Rectus Femoris
(The only muscle in the quadriceps group
to cross both the knee and hip joints)

Origin	Insertion	Action
Anterior inferior iliac spine and upper margin of the acetabulum	Patella and via the patellar ligament to the tibial tuberosity	Extends the knee and assists hip flexion

Vastus Medialis, Lateralis, and Intermedius

Origin	Insertion	Action
Vastus medialis and lateralis: linea aspera of the posterior femur Vastus intermedius: anterior and lateral shaft of the femur	Patella and via the patellar ligament to the tibial tuberosity	Knee extension

Functional Assessment

Range of motion: The quads extend the knee.

• The stretcher is seated, with legs dangling over the edge of the table. As the stretcher straightens the leg, the arc of motion should be smooth, and the knee should extend to 0° or beyond into a few degrees of hyperextension (Figure 3.8, a and b).

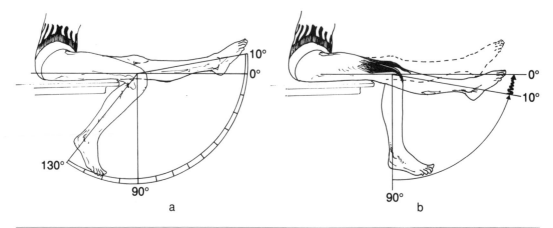

Figure 3.8   Normal range of knee extension: (a) The quadriceps should fully extend the knee. (b) The arc of motion should be smooth, with no hesitation or jerking.

• While on his stomach, the stretcher should be able to bring the heel to the buttock, with a little help from you (Figure 3.9). If range is limited, this may be due to tight quads, which will be somewhat uncomfortable as you press the heel toward the buttock, or limitation may be due to the bulk of the calf and hamstring muscles. PNF stretching works quite well here if the limitation is tight quads.

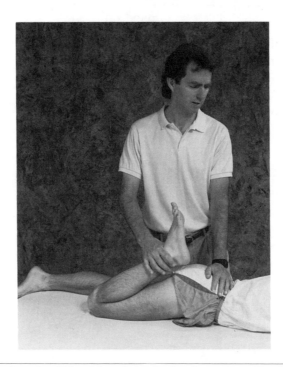

Figure 3.9   The stretcher should be able to bring heel to buttocks with a little help.

Instruction

1. The stretcher lies prone, with knee flexed as far as possible (Figure 3.10). This lengthens the quads to their end of range.

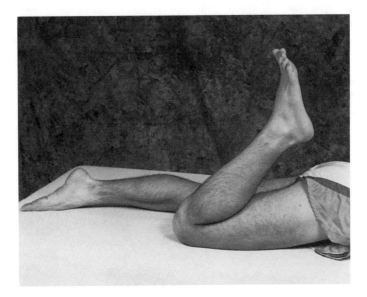

Figure 3.10   Initiation of the quadriceps stretch with the stretcher prone and knee flexed fully without help.

2. Offer resistance to the isometric contraction (no movement) of the quads by placing your hand or shoulder against the stretcher's shin (Figure 3.11, a and b).

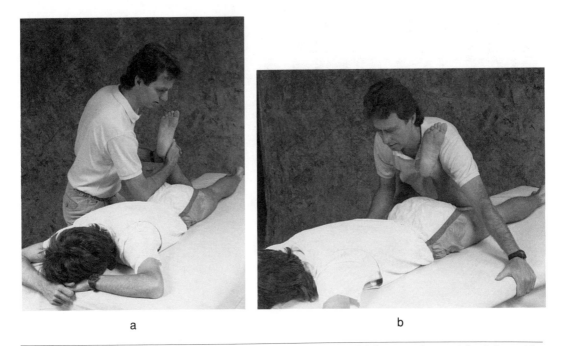

a   b

Figure 3.11   Offering resistance to the isometric contraction: (a) Support the stretcher's leg with your hands. (b) Support the stretcher's leg with your shoulder.

3. The stretcher tries to straighten his leg, isometrically contracting the quads, for 6 s. The stretcher begins slowly and builds to 50% to 100% of maximum contraction, breathing throughout.

4. The stretcher relaxes, breathes deeply, then contracts the hamstring, deepening the quad stretch. Occasionally the hamstring will go into spasm at this point, possibly because it is contracting from a new, shortened position. Stretching the hamstring prior to the quads usually prevents this problem.

5. Repeat 3 to 5 times.

6. *This is one of the few PNF stretches where you may push gently to assist the stretch.* After the second round of stretching, you may gently push the heel toward the buttock to help overcome the fleshy resistance of the calf and hamstring contact.

Stretching should be pain-free. If the stretcher experiences pain, reposition the leg, or use less force during the isometric contraction. If pain persists, don't use PNF until you know the cause of the pain.

Self-Stretching

The stretcher assumes the same beginning position as in instruction No. 1. The stretcher uses the opposite hand to hold the leg and provide resistance (right hand to left leg, left hand to right leg). This prevents excessive stress on the medial collateral ligament (Figure 3.12a). The stretcher may also use a towel wrapped around the leg if this is easier (Figure 3.12b).

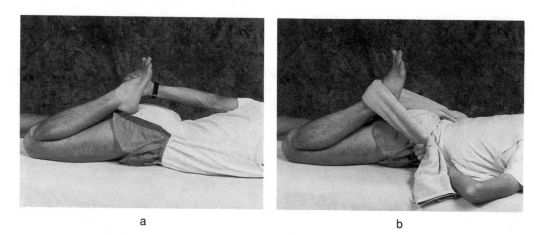

a   b

Figure 3.12   Quadriceps self-stretching: (a) The stretcher holds his leg with his opposite arm. (b) Self-stretching using a towel.

TIBIALIS ANTERIOR

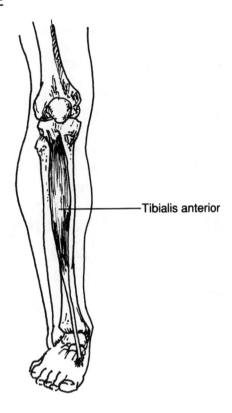

Tibialis anterior

Origin	Insertion	Action
Lateral shaft of the tibia, interosseous membrane	Base of the first metatarsal, first cuneiform	Ankle dorsiflexion, inversion of the foot

Functional Assessment

Check range of motion (Figure 3.13). Plantarflexion of the ankle should be approximately 50°. Dorsiflexion of the ankle should be approximately 20°. If range of motion is limited, PNF stretching may be helpful.

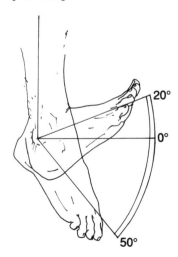

Figure 3.13   Normal range of plantarflexion and dorsiflexion of the ankle.

Instruction

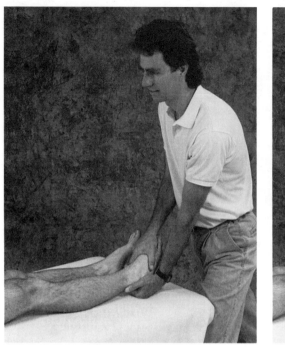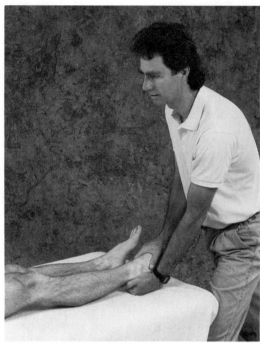

a   b

Figure 3.14   The initiation phase of the tibialis anterior stretch (right foot): (a) Provide resistance. Cup the stretcher's heel with your left hand and hold the top of the foot with your right hand. (b) The stretcher deepens the stretch.

1. The stretcher lies supine and plantarflexes the ankle (points toes) using the calf muscles. This lengthens the tibialis anterior to its end of range.

2. Grip the right heel with your left hand and the top of the foot with your right (Figure 3.14a) to offer resistance to the isometric contraction of the tibialis anterior. When stretching the left side, reverse your hand positions.

3. The stretcher pulls the foot toward the knee (dorsiflexion), isometrically contracting the tibialis anterior, for 6 s. The stretcher begins slowly and builds to 50% to 100% of maximum contraction, breathing throughout.

4. The stretcher relaxes, breathes deeply, then contracts the calf muscles to increase plantarflexion, deepening the tibialis anterior stretch (Figure 3.14b). *Never push to deepen the stretch.*

5. Repeat 3 to 5 times.

> **Stretching should be pain-free. If the stretcher experiences pain, reposition the foot, or use less force during the isometric contraction. If pain persists, don't use PNF until you know the cause of the pain.**

Self-Stretching

The stretcher follows the preceding steps, except to anchor the foot under a couch, a bed, or the strap of a sit-up bench to provide resistance to the isometric contraction.

PSOAS MAJOR AND ILIACUS

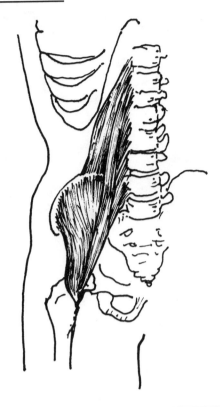

Origin	Insertion	Action
Psoas: anterior lumbar vertebrae Iliacus: inner surface of the ilium	Lesser trochanter of the femur	Flexion, adduction, and lateral rotation of the hip

Functional Assessment

Check range of motion. Normal range of flexion (120°) allows the stretcher to bring the flexed knee to the chest (Figure 3.15a). Normal range in extension is approximately 30° (Figure 3.15b).

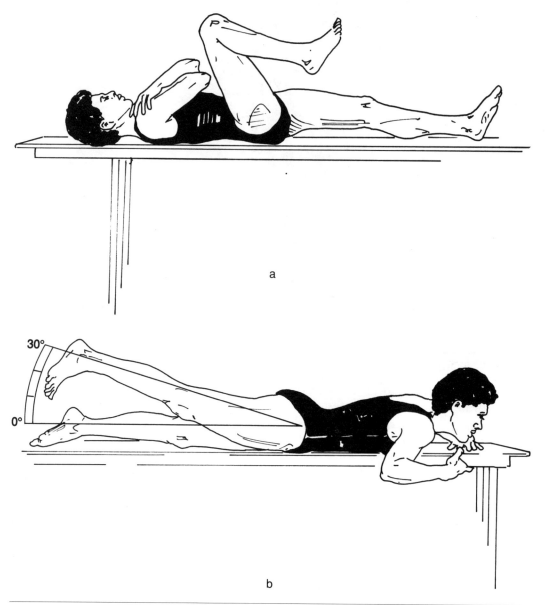

a

b

Figure 3.15   Normal range of hip (a) flexion and (b) extension.

To check for tightness in the psoas or quads, the stretcher lies supine with the lower legs dangling off the edge of the table, then lifts the right leg, knee to chest (Figure 3.16a).

Check for the following:

• The stretcher's left lower leg straightens. This indicates tight quads (especially rectus femoris) and tensor fascia latae on the left leg.

• The stretcher's left thigh lifts off the table (Figure 3.16b). This indicates a tight psoas on the left leg.

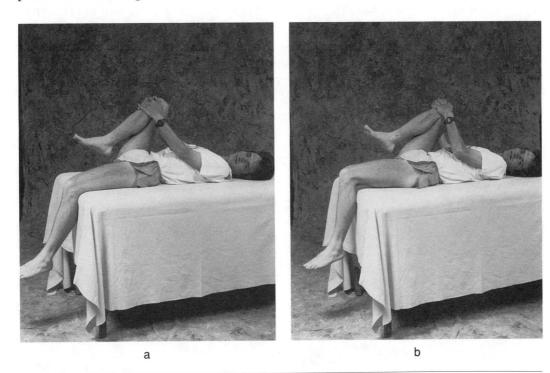

a   b

Figure 3.16   Testing for psoas and quadriceps tightness. (a) The stretcher flexes his right hip and knee, bringing the knee to his chest. The left leg extends, indicating a tight quadriceps, and possibly a tight tensor fascia latae, on the left. (b) His left thigh lifts off the table, indicating a tight psoas on the left.

Repeat for the other leg. It's common for both the quads and the psoas to be hypertonic on the same leg. If the psoas is tight, do PNF stretching for the psoas. If the quads are too tight, do PNF stretching for the quads.

Special Notes and Cautions

The iliopsoas is the major hip flexor. Because of its attachment along the lumbar spine, it affects the angle of the lumbar curve. If the psoas is too tight, it can increase the curve, which leads to swayback and low back pain. Conversely, sometimes a hypertonic psoas will straighten the lumbar curve, which also leads to low back pain.

Instruction

1. The stretcher lies supine with the greater trochanter of the femur at the edge of the table. This prevents limitation of hip extension by the table.

2. The stretcher lifts his right knee to his chest. This prevents extreme lordosis. (This is to protect the low back, especially in people with a history of low back pain.) The stretcher presses his left heel toward the floor, using the hip extensors (gluteals and hamstrings). This lengthens the left psoas to its end of range.

3. Offer resistance to the isometric contraction of the psoas by applying pressure with your right hand just above the left knee. Allow the stretcher to rest his right foot against you (Figure 3.17).

4. The stretcher pulls his left knee toward his left shoulder, isometrically contracting the psoas, for 6 s. The stretcher begins slowly and builds to 50% to 100% of maximum contraction, breathing throughout.

5. The stretcher relaxes, breathes deeply, then contracts the hip extensors (gluteals and hams) to press his left heel toward the floor, deepening the psoas stretch (Figure 3.18). *Never push to deepen the stretch.*

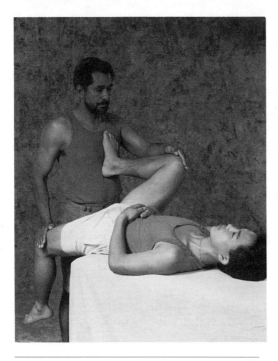

Figure 3.17   Initiation phase for stretching the left psoas. The greater trochanter is off the edge of the table.

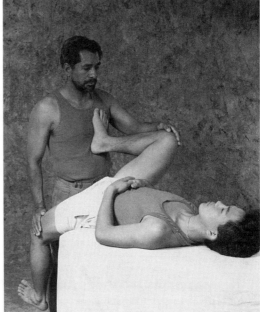

Figure 3.18   The stretcher actively deepens the stretch.

6. Repeat 3 to 5 times.

7. The stretcher may attempt to recruit his adductors by swinging the left leg into abduction and external rotation (Figure 3.19). Do not allow this.

8. To avoid extreme lordosis and possible low back pain, when you finish stretching the left side, help the stretcher bring both knees to his chest, then lower the right leg to stretch the right psoas. When both sides are finished, help the stretcher bring both knees to his chest. The stretcher then pushes himself more fully onto the table by pushing against you with both feet (Figure 3.20), then sits up carefully.

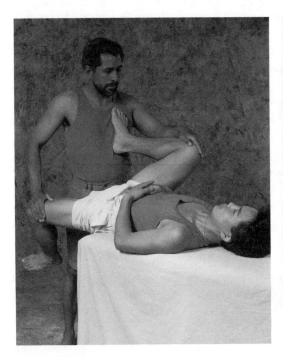

Figure 3.19 The stretcher's left leg is abducted and externally rotated in an attempt to recruit the adductors.

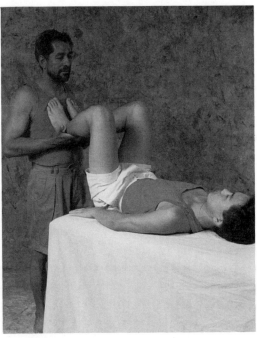

Figure 3.20 The stretcher pushes against you to slide further onto the table before sitting up.

Stretching should be pain-free. If the stretcher experiences pain, reposition the leg, or use less force during the isometric contraction. If pain persists, don't use PNF until you know the cause of the pain.

Self-Stretching

Although it's not a true PNF stretch, the following technique does take advantage of reciprocal inhibition to help stretch the psoas.

1. The stretcher takes the position in Figure 3.17, but supports his right leg with both of his own hands.

2. The stretcher allows the weight of the left leg to lengthen the psoas, for 10 to 20 s, then presses the left heel to the floor using the hip extensors.

3. Repeat 3 to 5 times.

Alternative instruction

1. The stretcher lies prone.

2. Stabilize the stretcher across the sacrum to keep his hips from lifting off the table.

3. The stretcher uses the hip extensors (gluteals and hamstrings) to lift his leg off the table as high as possible, with the knee bent. This lengthens the psoas to its end of range.

4. Support the leg just above the knee to provide resistance to the isometric contraction of the psoas. Use your hand or your leg to support the stretcher (Figure 3.21, a and b).

5. The stretcher pulls his thigh toward the table, isometrically contracting the psoas, for 6 s. The stretcher begins slowly and builds to 50% to 100% of maximum contraction, breathing throughout.

6. The stretcher relaxes, breathes deeply, then contracts the hip extensors to lift his thigh higher, deepening the psoas stretch. Continue to stabilize the hips to prevent them from lifting off the table. *Never pull to deepen the stretch.*

7. Repeat 3 to 5 times.

8. If you use your leg to provide resistance, move it closer to the hip with each round of stretching (Figure 3.21c).

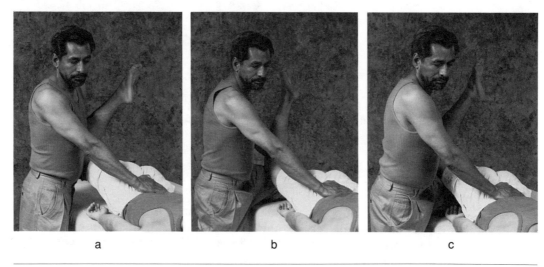

a   b   c

Figure 3.21   The initiation phase of the alternate psoas stretch: (a) Stabilize the stretcher's sacrum to keep hips on the table, and hold the stretcher's right leg with your left hand. (b) Support the stretcher's right leg with your thigh. (c) Move your thigh into a new support position.

Stretching should be pain-free. If the stretcher experiences pain, reposition the leg, or use less force during the isometric contraction. If pain persists, don't use PNF until you know the cause of the pain.

SOLEUS—GASTROCNEMIUS

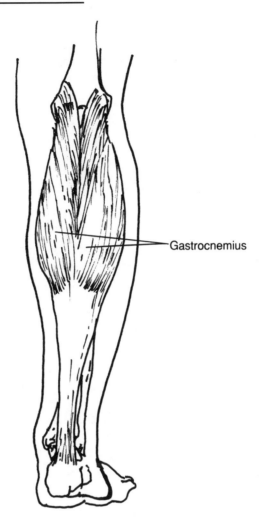

Gastrocnemius

Gastrocnemius

Origin	Insertion	Action
Medial head: medial epicondyle of the femur Lateral head: lateral epicondyle of the femur	Calcaneus via the Achilles tendon	Plantarflexion of the ankle or assists flexion of the knee, but it cannot do both simultaneously

Soleus

Origin	Insertion	Action
Soleal line of the tibia and posterior head and upper shaft of the fibula	Calcaneus via the Achilles tendon	Plantarflexion of the ankle (a stronger plantarflexor than the gastrocnemius)

Functional Assessment

Check range of motion.

• Dorsiflexion should be 20° (Figure 3.22a). If dorsiflexion is limited, have the stretcher lie prone and flex the knee to 90° and test again (Figure 3.22b). Knee flexion relaxes the gastrocnemius and eliminates it as a limiter of dorsiflexion.

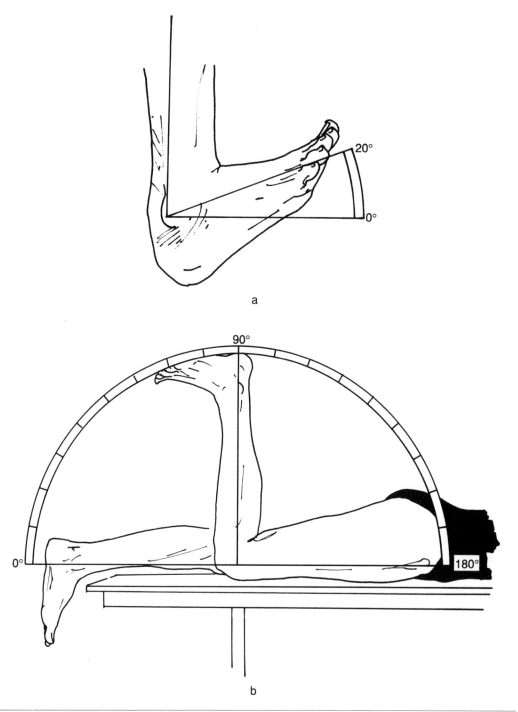

Figure 3.22   (a) Normal range of dorsiflexion of the ankle. (b) Dorsiflexion with the stretcher prone, knee flexed to 90°.

• Plantarflexion should be 50° (Figure 3.23). Limited plantarflexion may be due to a tight tibialis anterior.

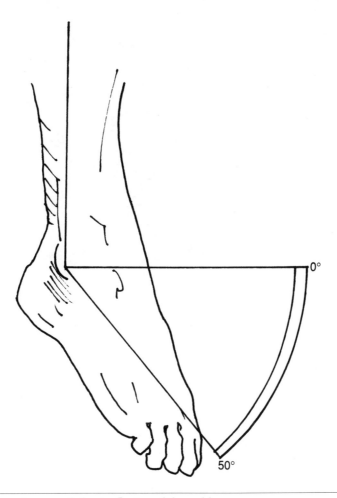

Figure 3.23   Normal range of plantarflexion of the ankle.

Instruction

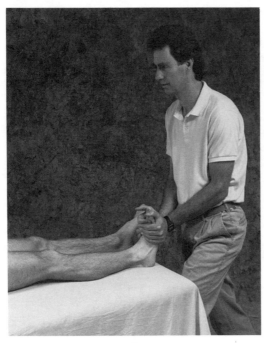
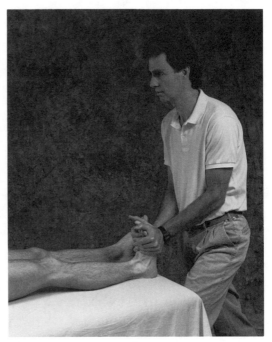

a   b

Figure 3.24   Initiation phase of the gastrocnemius/soleus stretch: (a) Assume a wide stance and resist with both hands. (b) The stretcher actively deepens the stretch.

1. The stretcher lies supine and grips the sides of the table to keep from sliding during the isometric phase.

2. The stretcher dorsiflexes his foot as far as possible. This lengthens the gastrocnemius/soleus to its end of range.

3. Offer resistance to the isometric contraction of the gastrocnemius/soleus by standing at the end of the table and placing both hands around the foot and using your body weight to prevent plantarflexion (Figure 3.24a).

4. The stretcher tries to point his foot (plantarflex), isometrically contracting the gastrocnemius/soleus, for 6 s. The stretcher begins slowly and builds to 50% to 100% of maximum contraction, breathing throughout.

5. The stretcher relaxes, breathes deeply, then contracts the tibialis anterior, deepening the gastrocnemius/soleus stretch (Figure 3.24b). *Never push to deepen the stretch*.

6. Repeat 3 to 5 times.

Stretching should be pain-free. If the stretcher experiences pain, reposition the leg or foot, or use less force during the isometric contraction. If pain persists, don't use PNF until you know the cause of the pain.

Self-Stretching

For this muscle group, self-stretching probably works better than partner-assisted stretching. The technique is the same, except that the stretcher sits with the leg extended, a towel wrapped around the foot and held in both hands to provide resistance during the isometric phase (Figure 3.25).

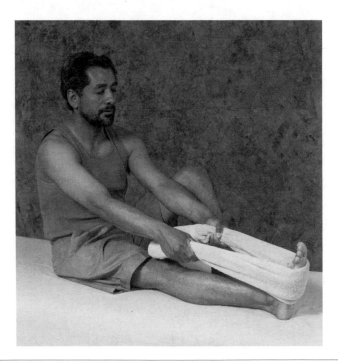

Figure 3.25   Self-stretching using a towel.

Adductors

The adductor muscles can be divided into short adductors and long adductors. The two groups will be treated separately in the following stretches.

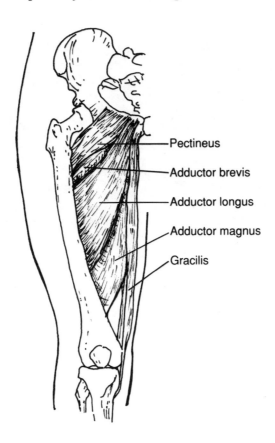

SHORT ADDUCTORS

Pectineus

Origin	Insertion	Action
Anterior pubis	Between the lesser trochanter and the linea aspera of the posterior femur	Hip flexion, assists adduction and lateral rotation of the hip

Adductor Longus and Brevis

Origin	Insertion	Action
Anterior pubis	Linea aspera of the posterior femur	Adduction of hip, assists flexion and lateral rotation of the hip

LONG ADDUCTORS

Adductor Magnus

Origin	Insertion	Action
Pubic ramus, ischial tuberosity	Linea aspera of the posterior femur, adductor tubercle of the medial femur	Powerful adduction of hip The anterior fibers (origin on pubic ramus) assist hip flexion The posterior fibers (origin on ischial tuberosity) assist hip extension

Gracilis

Origin	Insertion	Action
Anterior pubis	Medial proximal tibia (pes anserine)	Adduction of the hip, assists knee flexion and medial rotation of the leg with the knee flexed

Functional Assessment

Check the range of motion. Normally, the legs should be able to open 45° to 50° from the midline (Figure 3.26). If this range is limited, it's often due to tight adductors. Use PNF stretching to increase this range.

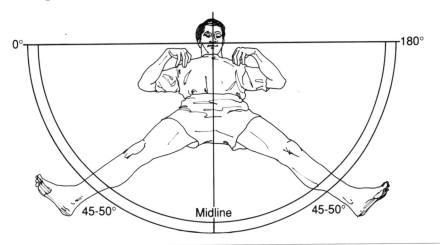

Figure 3.26   Normal range of abduction of the legs. If this is limited, it's probably due to tight adductors.

Special Notes and Cautions

The adductors assist hip flexion and help to stabilize the legs in running. They are commonly much tighter in men. Groin pulls are often related to fatigue or improper stretching of the adductor longus.

Instruction—Short Adductors

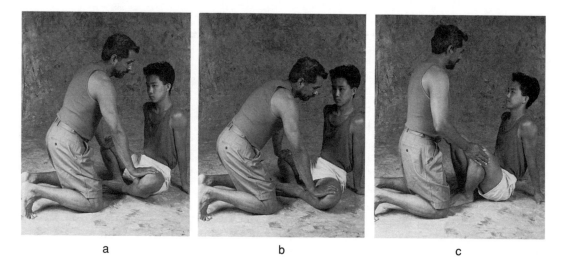

a   b   c

Figure 3.27   (a) Initiation phase of the short adductors stretch. (b) The stretcher actively deepens the stretch. (c) Assist the stretcher in bringing legs together after the stretch.

1. The stretcher is seated, with the knees bent and the soles of the feet together.

2. The stretcher pulls his knees toward the floor, using the hip abductors (gluteus medius and minimus). This lengthens the short adductors to their end of range.

3. Place your hands on the stretcher's medial knees (Figure 3.27a) to provide resistance to the isometric contraction of the adductors.

4. The stretcher tries to pull his knees together, isometrically contracting the short adductors, for 6 s. The stretcher begins slowly and builds to 50% to 100% of maximum contraction, breathing throughout.

5. The stretcher relaxes, breathes deeply, then contracts the hip abductors to pull his knees toward the floor (Figure 3.27b). This deepens the adductor stretch. *Never push to deepen the stretch.*

6. Repeat 3 to 5 times.

7. After the final stretch, help the stretcher bring his knees together to avoid groin strain from this vulnerable position (Figure 3.27c).

8. The stretcher will sometimes get abductor cramps during this stretch. It's helpful to stretch the abductors first.

Stretching should be pain-free. If the stretcher experiences pain, reposition the legs, or use less force during the isometric contraction. If pain persists, don't use PNF until you know the cause of the pain.

Instruction—Long Adductors

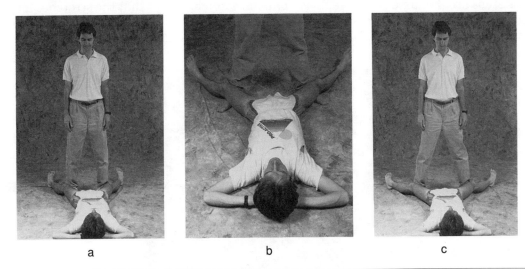

a   b   c

Figure 3.28 (a) Initiation phase of the long adductors stretch. (b) An alternate position, with your bare feet under the stretcher's knees. (c) The stretcher actively deepens the stretch.

1. The stretcher lies supine on the floor, his legs straight, with no hip rotation (the kneecaps pointed toward the ceiling) to avoid stretching the hamstrings.

2. The stretcher spreads his legs as far as possible, using the hip abductors (gluteus medius and minimus). This lengthens the adductors to their end of range.

3. Stand between the stretcher's legs and place your feet just proximal to the stretcher's knees (Figure 3.28a) to provide resistance to the isometric contraction of the adductors. Resistance is given just above the knee to avoid straining the medial collateral ligaments. An optional position is to place your feet diagonally under the stretcher's knees (Figure 3.28b). This may be more comfortable and secure for both of you.

4. The stretcher tries to pull the knees together, isometrically contracting the adductors, for 6 s. The stretcher begins slowly and builds to 50% to 100% of maximum contraction, breathing throughout.

5. The stretcher relaxes, breathes deeply, then contracts the hip abductors to pull the legs farther apart (Figure 3.28c). This deepens the adductor stretch. *Never push to deepen the stretch*.

6. Repeat 3 to 5 times.

7. After the final stretch, help the stretcher bring his legs together to avoid groin strain from this vulnerable position.

8. The stretcher will sometimes get abductor cramps during this stretch. It's helpful to stretch the abductors first.

Stretching should be pain-free. If the stretcher experiences pain, reposition the legs, or use less force during the isometric contraction. If pain persists, don't use PNF until you know the cause of the pain.

Self-Stretching

The steps are the same as for the short adductor stretch, except that the stretcher uses his own arms to provide resistance against the medial knees during the isometric contraction (Figure 3.29). *The stretcher should never push to deepen the stretch.*

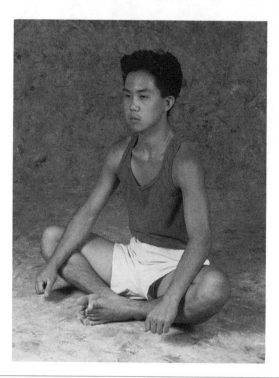

Figure 3.29 Self-stretching for the short adductors.

TENSOR FASCIA LATAE AND IT BAND

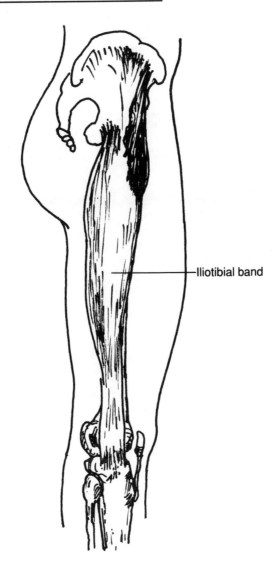

Iliotibial band

Tensor Fascia Latae (TFL)

Origin	Insertion	Action
Iliac crest, just posterior to the anterior superior iliac spine	Iliotibial band, which inserts at the lateral tibial condyle (Gerdy's tubercle)	Prevents the knee from collapsing during movement. Assists abduction, medial rotation, and flexion of the hip. Assists knee extension

Functional Assessment

The TFL and IT band function primarily as knee stabilizers. Problems develop when the TFL is hypertonic (too tight). To test for this, have the stretcher lying on his side, with the knee of the top leg tucked behind the knee of the other leg (Figure 3.30). Excessive tightness in the TFL prevents this position and can lead to other problems, such as IT band syndrome.

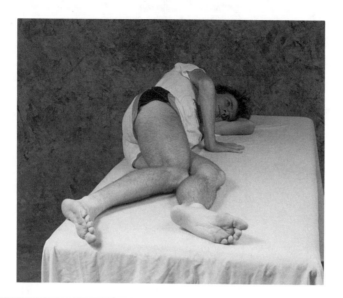

Figure 3.30   Tensor fascia latae tightness test.

Special Notes and Cautions

IT band syndrome is an overuse injury caused by a tight IT band rubbing over the lateral femoral condyle. The syndrome is often found in cyclists and novice runners who overpronate. Pain is normally experienced just proximal to the lateral knee, but it may also be found at the IT band insertion on the tibia. Figure 3.31 shows the areas of pain. Tightness in the band can be caused by a tight TFL, which pulls on the band, or by a hypertrophied vastus lateralis, which bulges under the band and stretches it.

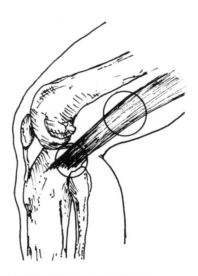

Figure 3.31   Iliotibial band syndrome pain sites.

Instruction

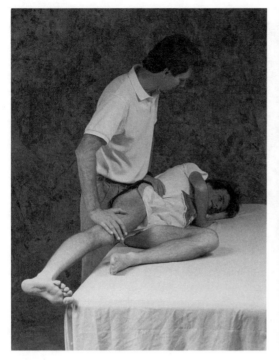
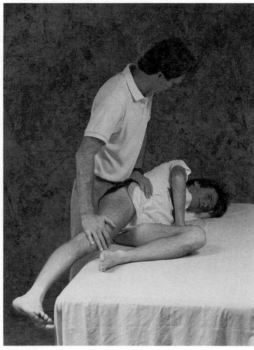

a   b

Figure 3.32   (a) Initiation phase of the tensor fascia latae stretch. (b) The stretcher actively deepens the stretch.

1. The stretcher is lying on his side with his back at the edge of the table, top leg hyperextended and hanging over the edge of the table. The stretcher contracts his adductors to pull the leg toward the floor, lengthening the TFL to its end of range.

2. Stand behind the stretcher to offer support, and stabilize his hip with one hand. With the other hand, offer resistance just above the knee to the isometric contraction of the TFL (Figure 3.32a).

3. The stretcher tries to abduct the hip, isometrically contracting the TFL, for 6 s. The stretcher begins slowly and builds to 50% to 100% of maximum contraction, breathing throughout.

4. The stretcher relaxes, breathes deeply, then contracts the adductors, deepening the TFL stretch (Figure 3.32b). *Never push to deepen the stretch.*

5. Repeat 3 to 5 times.

Stretching should be pain-free. If the stretcher experiences pain, reposition the leg, or use less force during the isometric contraction. If pain persists, don't use PNF until you know the cause of the pain.

If the stretcher is too strong for you to offer effective resistance, a towel may be used to provide resistance to the isometric contraction (Figure 3.33).

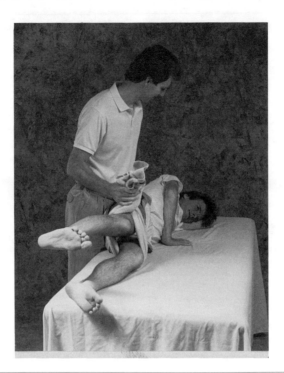

Figure 3.33   Using a towel to provide resistance.

Alternative Instruction

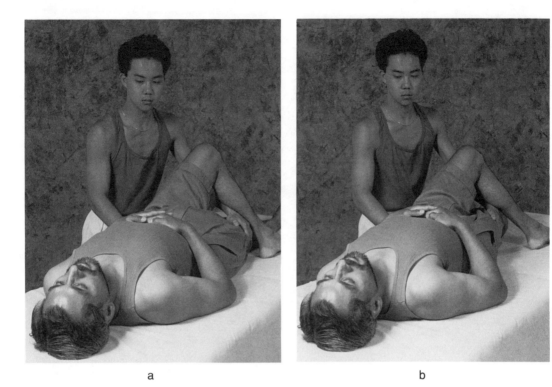

a   b

Figure 3.34   (a) Initiation phase of the alternate tensor fascia latae stretch. (b) The stretcher actively deepens the stretch.

1. The stretcher lies supine, with the target leg straight and the other leg placed over the target leg, with the knee bent and the foot flat on the table. The stretcher adducts the target leg across the midline as far as possible, lengthening the TFL to its end range.

2. Offer resistance just above the knee to the isometric contraction of the TFL (Figure 3.34a).

3. The stretcher tries to abduct his hip, isometrically contracting the TFL, for 6 s. The stretcher begins slowly and builds to 50% to 100% of maximum contraction, breathing throughout.

4. The stretcher relaxes, breathes deeply, then contracts the adductors, deepening the TFL stretch (Figure 3.34b). *Never pull to deepen the stretch.*

5. Repeat 3 to 5 times.

Stretching should be pain-free. If the stretcher experiences pain, reposition the leg, or use less force during the isometric contraction. If pain persists, don't use PNF until you know the cause of the pain.

PIRIFORMIS

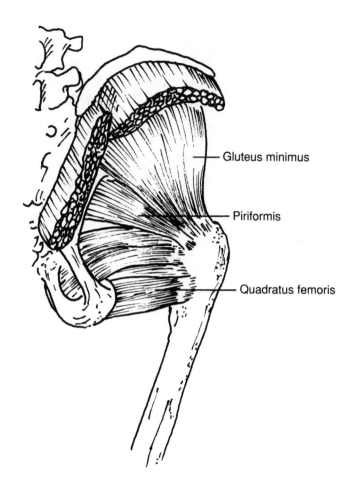

- Gluteus minimus
- Piriformis
- Quadratus femoris

Origin	Insertion	Action
Anterior sacrum	Superior aspect of the greater trochanter	Lateral rotation of the femur, assists abduction of the femur

Functional Assessment

The piriformis is one of six deep lateral hip rotators, all of which insert on some portion of the greater trochanter. When these muscles are hypertonic, they contribute to a toe-out gait, commonly seen in dancers, and they restrict internal rotation of the hip. Stretching the piriformis also stretches the other lateral rotators.

Special Notes and Cautions

Tightness in the lateral rotators, of which the piriformis is one, is a common cause of sciatic pain. The sciatic nerve exits the sciatic notch of the ilium and travels through these muscles on its way to the posterior thigh (Figure 3.35). When the muscles are hypertonic, they can squeeze the nerve, causing irritation and pain. You can differentiate this type of sciatica (known as piriformis syndrome) from true sciatica by determining where the pain begins. If shooting or burning pain begins at the lumbar spine and travels down the leg, then it is likely to be true sciatica. If this type of pain begins in the buttocks, it's probably due to piriformis syndrome and responds well to massage and stretching.

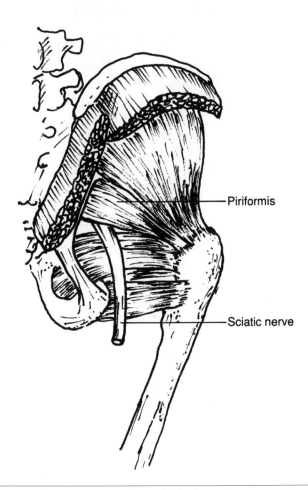

Figure 3.35 The path of the sciatic nerve through the lateral rotators.

Instruction

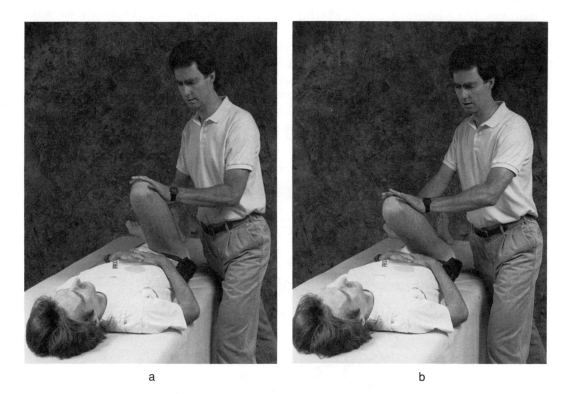

a   b

Figure 3.36   (a) Initiation phase of the piriformis stretch. (b) The stretcher actively deepens the stretch.

1. The stretcher lies supine, with the hip and knee flexed and drawn up toward the opposite shoulder; the other leg is straight. This lengthens the piriformis to its comfortable end range.

2. Place both your hands on the stretcher's lateral knee (Figure 3.36a) to offer resistance to the isometric contraction.

3. The stretcher pushes his knee diagonally toward you, isometrically contracting the piriformis, for 6 s. The stretcher starts slowly and builds to 50% to 100% of maximum contraction, breathing throughout.

4. The stretcher relaxes, breathes deeply, and contracts his hip flexors and adductors to deepen the piriformis stretch (Figure 3.36b). You may assist by *gently* pushing to deepen the stretch.

5. Repeat 3 to 5 times.

Stretching should be pain-free. If the stretcher experiences pain, reposition the leg, or use less force during the isometric contraction. If pain persists, don't use PNF until you know the cause of the pain.

Self-Stretching

The stretcher assumes the same beginning position, and uses his own hands to provide resistance (Figure 3.37).

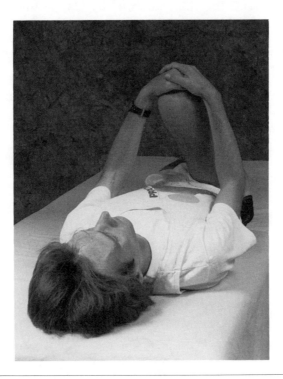

Figure 3.37   Piriformis self-stretch.

STRETCHES FOR THE UPPER EXTREMITIES

This section covers the muscles of the shoulder, arm, and wrist. I've grouped the four muscles of the rotator cuff together, followed by the pectoralis. These muscles all provide motion at the shoulder.

The format of this section is designed to provide you with the information you need to use PNF most effectively. Please be sure to read the special notes and cautions before doing any stretching. Each section is presented as follows:

- Origin, insertion, and action of muscle(s), with illustration
- Functional assessment for normal range of motion
- Special notes and cautions
- Detailed stretching instructions, with illustrations
- Self-stretching instructions, where appropriate, with illustrations
- Alternative stretching instructions, where appropriate, with illustrations

ROTATOR CUFF MUSCLES

The tendons of four muscles form the rotator cuff and stabilize the humerus in the glenoid fossa of the scapula during movement.

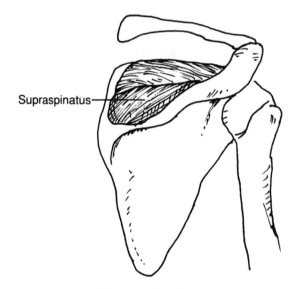

Supraspinatus

Supraspinatus

Origin	Insertion	Action
Supraspinous fossa of the scapula	Greater tubercle of the humerus (superior facet)	Stabilizes the head of the humerus to initiate abduction

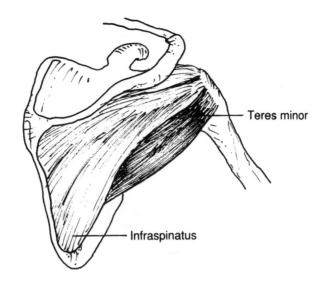

Infraspinatus

Origin	Insertion	Action
Infraspinous fossa of the scapula	Greater tubercle of the humerus (middle facet)	Lateral rotation of the humerus

Teres Minor

Origin	Insertion	Action
Upper axillary border of the scapula	Greater tubercle of the humerus (inferior facet)	Lateral rotation of the humerus

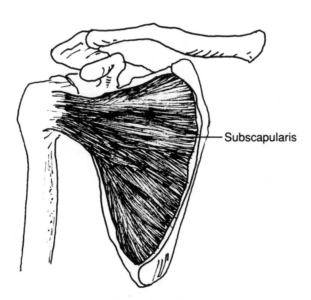

Subscapularis

Origin	Insertion	Action
Subscapularis fossa of the scapula	Lesser tubercle of the humerus	Medial rotation of the humerus

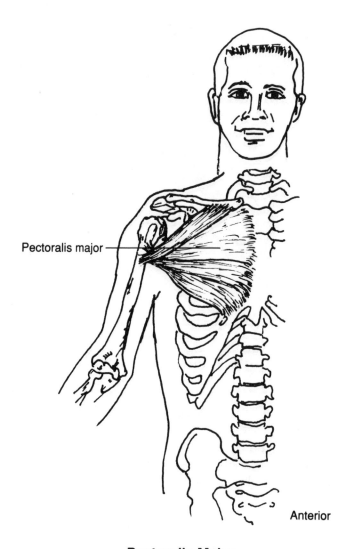

Pectoralis major

Anterior

Pectoralis Major

Origin	Insertion	Action
Clavicular head: Medial half of the clavicle Sternal head: Sternum and cartilage of the six upper ribs	Lateral lip of the bicipital groove of the humerus	Adduction, horizontal adduction, and medial rotation of the humerus Clavicular head: Flexion of the humerus Sternal head: Extension of the humerus from a flexed position

Functional Assessment

Active range of motion: The shoulder joint has the greatest range of motion of any joint in the body. Active movements can be used to evaluate the entire shoulder complex (humerus, clavicle, scapula) for freedom of movement and for pain.

Refer to Figures 3.38, a-d for the normal ranges of shoulder motion:

Internal rotation = 90°	Flexion = 180°
External rotation = 50°	Extension = 60°
Horizontal adduction = 130°	Adduction = 45°
Horizontal abduction = 30°	Abduction = 180°

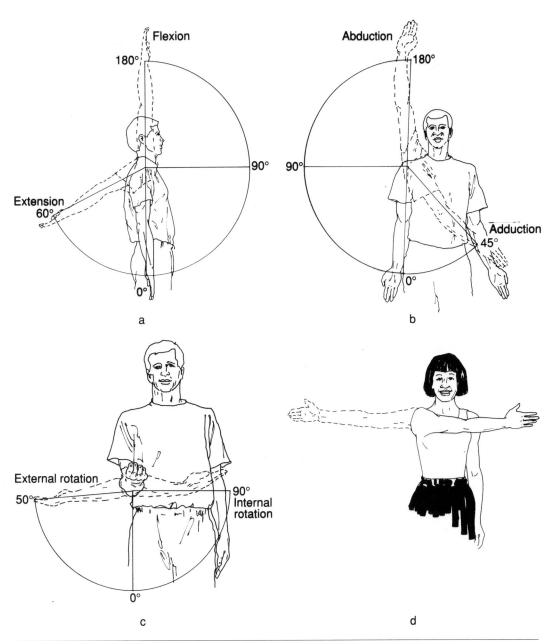

Figure 3.38   (a) Normal shoulder flexion-extension. (b) Normal shoulder adduction-abduction. (c) Normal shoulder internal and external rotation. (d) Normal shoulder horizontal adduction-abduction.

Instruction—Rotator Cuff Muscles

If range of motion is normal in the shoulder, PNF stretching for flexibility is unnecessary. It is useful, however, to soften hypertonic muscles prior to trigger-point work or deep massage. I've listed the typical PNF stretches here. You can improvise others as needed.

Subscapularis

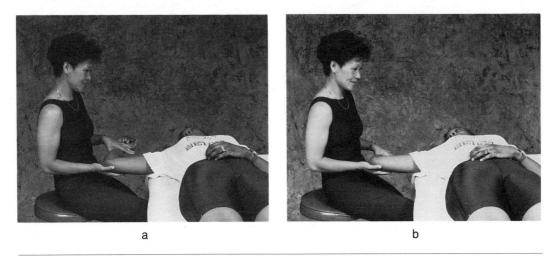

a   b

Figure 3.39 Initiation phase of the subscapularis stretch: (a) Resist and stabilize the stretcher's arm; (b) the stretcher actively deepens the stretch.

1. The stretcher lies supine with her shoulder at the edge of the table. Her elbow is flexed to 90°, and her arm is externally rotated as far as possible. This lengthens the subscapularis to its pain-free end of range.

2. Offer resistance to the isometric contraction of the subscapularis by stabilizing the elbow and wrist (Figure 3.39a).

3. The stretcher attempts to internally rotate the humerus, isometrically contracting the subscapularis, for 6 s. The stretcher begins slowly and builds to 50% to 100% of maximum contraction, breathing throughout.

4. The stretcher relaxes, breathes deeply, then contracts the infraspinatus, deepening the subscapularis stretch (Figure 3.39b). *Never push to deepen the stretch.*

5. Repeat 3 to 5 times.

Stretching should be pain-free. If the stretcher experiences pain, reposition the arm, or use less force during the isometric contraction. If pain persists, don't use PNF until you know the cause of the pain.

Infraspinatus

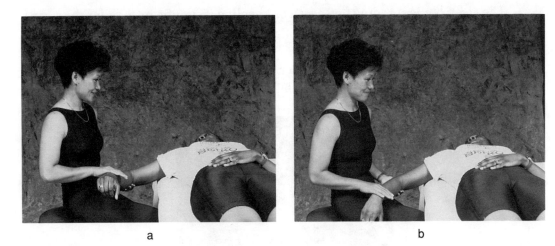

a   b

Figure 3.40   Initiation phase of the infraspinatus stretch: (a) Resist and stabilize the stretcher's arm; (b) the stretcher actively deepens the stretch.

1. The stretcher is in the same position as for the subscapularis stretch, except the humerus is internally rotated. This lengthens the infraspinatus to its pain-free end of range.

2. Offer resistance to the isometric contraction of the infraspinatus by stabilizing the elbow and wrist (Figure 3.40a).

3. The stretcher attempts external rotation of the humerus, isometrically contracting the infraspinatus, for 6 s. The stretcher begins slowly and builds to 50% to 100% of maximum contraction, breathing throughout.

4. The stretcher relaxes, breathes deeply, then contracts the subscapularis, deepening the infraspinatus stretch (Figure 3.40b). *Never push to deepen the stretch*.

5. Repeat 3 to 5 times.

Stretching should be pain-free. If the stretcher experiences pain, reposition the arm, or use less force during the isometric contraction. If pain persists, don't use PNF until you know the cause of the pain.

Instruction—Pectoralis

1. The stretcher is standing (or seated or kneeling if significantly taller than you).

2. Working bilaterally, the stretcher flexes, abducts, and externally rotates the humerus and flexes the elbow to 90°.

3. Position yourself behind the stretcher to stabilize and offer resistance during the isometric contraction of the pectoralis (Figure 3.41).

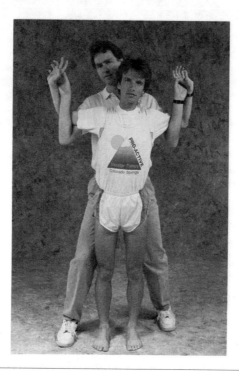

Figure 3.41   Initiation phase of the pectoralis stretch.

4. The stretcher attempts to adduct his arms horizontally, contracting pectoralis (and anterior deltoids) isometrically, for 6 s. The stretcher begins slowly, building to 50% to 100% of maximum contraction, breathing throughout.

5. The stretcher relaxes, breathes deeply, then contracts the horizontal abductors again, deepening the stretch on the pectoralis. *Never pull to deepen the stretch*.

6. Repeat 3 to 5 times.

Stretching should be pain-free. If the stretcher experiences pain, reposition the arms, or use less force during the isometric contraction. If pain persists, don't use PNF until you know the cause of the pain.

Self-Stretching

PNF stretching for the rotator cuff is difficult without a partner. The stretcher can use the positioning described for the subscapularis and the infraspinatus to do passive stretching, assisted by moderate weight (5 to 10 lb) to increase range of motion. The stretcher lies supine with the arm positioned in external or internal rotation, as in the beginning positions described for partner stretching. The stretcher holds the weight in the hand and lets gravity work for a minute or so while focusing on breathing deeply and relaxing the shoulder (Figure 3.42). An increase in flexibility should be noticeable.

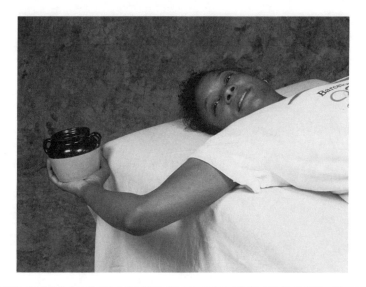

Figure 3.42   Self-stretch of the subscapularis.

Self-stretching of the pectoralis can be done using a doorway to provide resistance during the isometric phase (Figure 3.43). The arm is raised higher or lower to stretch different parts of the pectoralis.

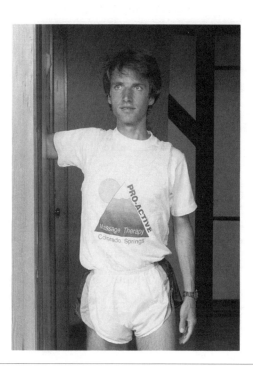

Figure 3.43   Self-stretch of the pectoralis using a doorway.

PRIMARY WRIST FLEXORS

Limited range of motion at the wrist is uncommon unless the wrist has been immobilized for some reason. Because the wrist muscles are used extensively in daily activity, even "leg-sport" athletes will benefit from stretching these muscles. Three primary muscles act to flex the wrist: flexor carpi radialis, flexor carpi ulnaris, and palmaris longus. Their common origin on the medial epicondyle is the site of "golfer's elbow," an overuse tendinitis.

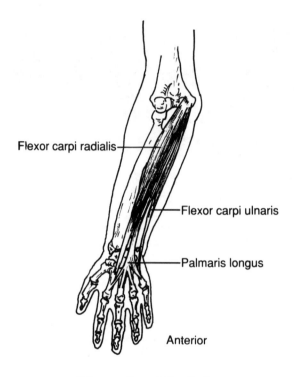

Flexor Carpi Radialis

Origin	Insertion	Action
Medial epicondyle of the humerus	Base of the 2nd and 3rd metacarpals	Flexion and abduction of the wrist

Flexor Carpi Ulnaris

Origin	Insertion	Action
Medial epicondyle of the humerus and the proximal posterior ulna	Pisiform, hamate, and base of the 5th metacarpal	Flexion and adduction of the wrist

Palmaris Longus (sometimes absent)

Origin	Insertion	Action
Medial epicondyle of the humerus	Palmar aponeurosis	Assists flexion of the wrist

PRIMARY WRIST EXTENSORS

There are also three primary muscles that extend the wrist: extensor carpi radialis longus, extensor carpi radialis brevis, and extensor carpi ulnaris. Their common origin on the lateral epicondyle is the primary site of "tennis elbow," an overuse tendinitis common in racket sports.

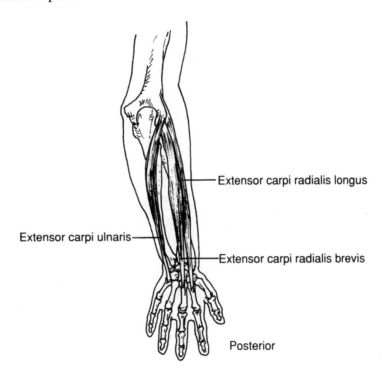

Extensor Carpi Radialis Longus

Origin	Insertion	Action
Lateral epicondyle and lateral supracondylar ridge of the humerus	Base of the 2nd metacarpal	Extension and abduction of the wrist

Extensor Carpi Radialis Brevis

Origin	Insertion	Action
Lateral epicondyle of the humerus	Base of the 3rd metacarpal	Extension of the wrist

Extensor Carpi Ulnaris

Origin	Insertion	Action
Lateral epicondyle of the humerus and posterior proximal ulna	Base of the 5th metacarpal	Extension and adduction of the wrist

Functional Assessment

Active range of motion: Measurements are taken from the wrist in neutral (Figures 3.44, a and b). Normal ranges are

flexion = 80°
extension = 70°
ulnar deviation (adduction) = 30°
radial deviation (abduction) = 20°

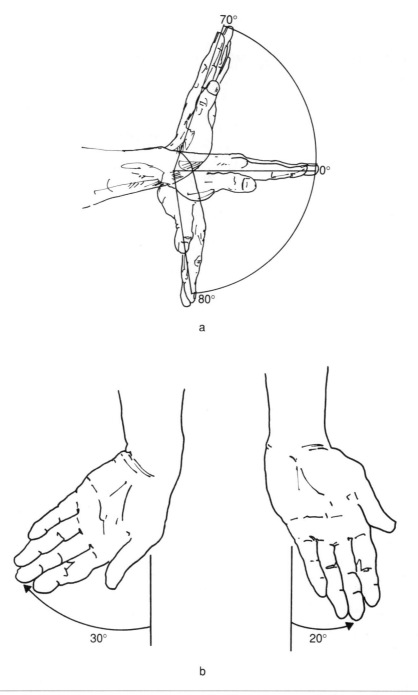

a

b

Figure 3.44 (a) Normal wrist flexion-extension. (b) Normal ulnar-radial deviation.

Special Notes and Cautions

PNF stretching can be used to soften the wrist muscles before massage or trigger-point work. Baseball players, racquetball players, musicians, grocery clerks, and typists are commonly afflicted with hypertonic wrist and forearm muscles. Regular PNF sessions can help reduce the risk of repetitive motion syndrome and overuse tendinitis.

Instruction—Wrist Flexors

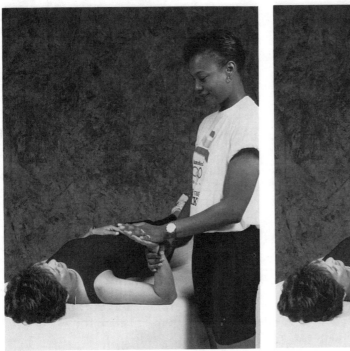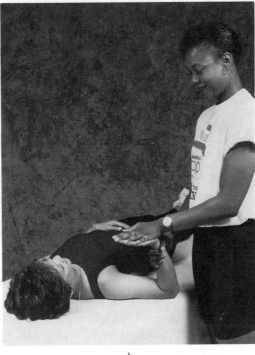

a   b

Figure 3.45   (a) Initiation phase for flexors. (b) Assist the stretcher in deepening the stretch.

1. The stretcher lies supine, with her elbow bent to approximately 90° and her wrist extended as far as possible with the fingers straight. This lengthens the flexors to their pain-free end of range.

2. Place the palm and fingers of one of your hands over the palm and fingers of the stretcher's hand. Your other hand stabilizes the stretcher's wrist and forearm (Figure 3.45a).

3. Offer resistance to the isometric contraction of the wrist and finger flexors.

4. The stretcher attempts to flex her fingers and wrist, isometrically contracting the flexors, for 6 s. The stretcher begins slowly and builds to 50% to 100% of maximum contraction, breathing throughout.

5. The stretcher relaxes, breathes deeply, then contracts the extensors, deepening the wrist flexor stretch (Figure 3.45b). You may *gently* assist to deepen the stretch by pushing on the stretcher's fingers.

6. Repeat 3 to 5 times.

Stretching should be pain-free. If the stretcher experiences pain, reposition the wrist and arm, or use less force during the isometric contraction. If pain persists, don't use PNF until you know the cause of the pain.

Instruction—Wrist Extensors

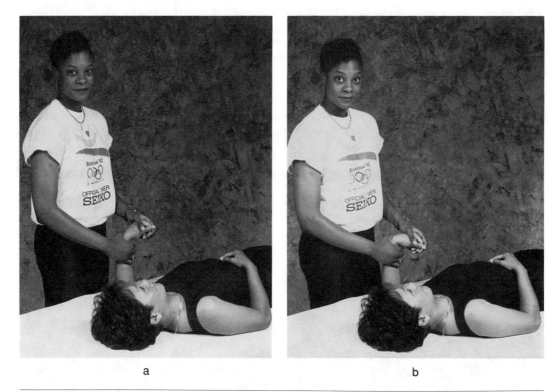

a   b

Figure 3.46 (a) Initiation phase for extensors. (b) Assist the stretcher in deepening the stretch.

1. The stretcher lies supine, with her elbow bent to approximately 90° and her wrist flexed as far as possible with the fingers rolled into a loose fist. This lengthens the wrist extensors to their pain-free end of range.

2. Wrap one hand over the stretcher's fist and use your other hand to stabilize the stretcher's forearm (Figure 3.46a).

3. Offer resistance to the isometric contraction of the wrist and finger extensors.

4. The stretcher attempts to extend her wrist and fingers, isometrically contracting the extensors, for 6 s. The stretcher starts slowly and builds to 50% to 100% of maximum contraction, breathing throughout.

5. The stretcher relaxes, breathes deeply, and contracts the wrist flexors to deepen the stretch (Figure 3.46b). You may *gently* push to deepen the stretch.

6. Repeat 3 to 5 times.

Stretching should be pain-free. If the stretcher experiences pain, reposition the wrist and arm, or use less force during the isometric contraction. If pain persists, don't use PNF until you know the cause of the pain.

Self-Stretching

The stretcher can provide isometric resistance for these stretches by using her other hand (Figure 3.47, a and b).

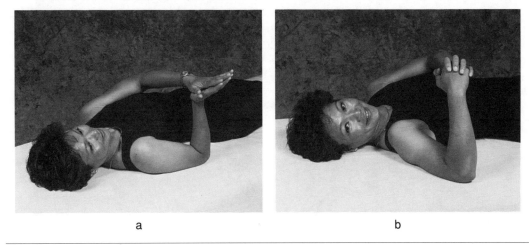

a   b

Figure 3.47   Self-stretch for (a) flexors and (b) extensors.

TRICEPS

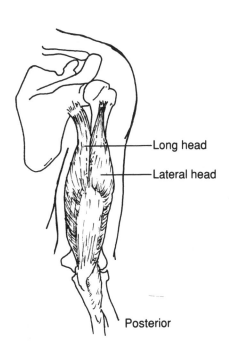

Origin	Insertion	Action
Long head: Infraglenoid tubercle of the scapula	Olecranon process of the ulna	Extension of the elbow
Lateral head: Posterolateral surface of the proximal humerus		Long head: extension of the humerus
Medial head: Lower two thirds of the postero-medial humerus		

Functional Assessment

The triceps, a three-headed, two-joint muscle, crosses both the shoulder and the elbow. Normal range of motion at the elbow is 135° or more for flexion and 0° for extension (Figure 3.48). Flexion may be limited by the muscle mass of the anterior arm or by a hypertonic triceps. Generally, the stretcher should be able to touch the front of her shoulder. Extension of the elbow may be limited by a hypertonic biceps. The triceps also extends the humerus and may limit full flexion if it is hypertonic.

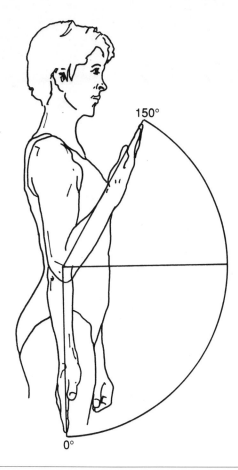

Figure 3.48   Normal flexion-extension of the elbow.

Instruction

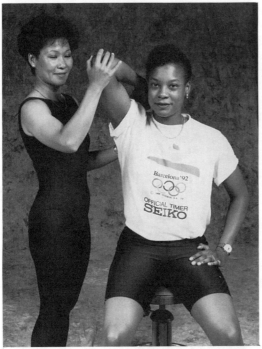
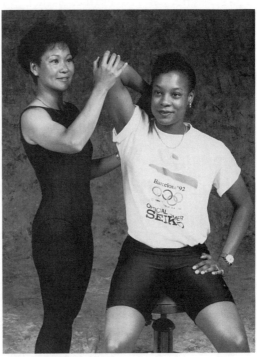

a   b

Figure 3.49 Initiation phase of triceps stretch: (a) Resist and stabilize while facing the stretcher; (b) the stretcher actively deepens the stretch.

1. The stretcher is seated, with her shoulder and elbow fully flexed. The elbow should be pointed toward the ceiling, and her hand should be flat against the back. This lengthens the tricep to its pain-free end of range.

2. Stand facing the stretcher, with one hand stabilizing at the scapula, the other on the upraised elbow, to offer resistance to the isometric contraction of the triceps and to ensure that the stretcher keeps her back straight (Figure 3.49a).

3. The stretcher attempts to extend the humerus (keeping the elbow flexed), isometrically contracting the triceps, for 6 s. The stretcher begins slowly, building to 50% to 100% of maximum, breathing throughout.

4. The stretcher relaxes, breathes deeply, and contracts her shoulder flexors to deepen the stretch (Figure 3.49b). *Never push to deepen the stretch.*

5. Repeat 3 to 5 times.

Stretching should be pain-free. If the stretcher experiences pain, reposition the arm, or use less force during the isometric contraction. If pain persists, don't use PNF until you know the cause of the pain.

Self-Stretching

The stretcher can provide isometric resistance for this stretch by using her other arm and hand (Figure 3.50). Erect posture must be maintained during this stretch to achieve the best results.

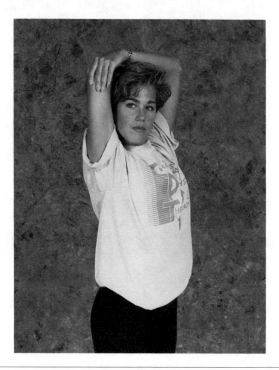

Figure 3.50   Emphasize good posture when self-stretching.

STRETCHES FOR THE TORSO

Torso muscles are primarily postural muscles. Our daily lives require a great deal of flexion in the torso and neck—we sit at desks, in cars, in front of the TV. Because our chairs are not designed to support our bodies well, the postural muscles are called on to take up the slack. Most sports also require a great deal of support and active involvement from the torso muscles. Almost everyone has excess tension in these muscles, so PNF techniques are a quick and simple way to provide more ease and comfort in these core areas. The following stretches can be used as preventive techniques or to help relieve pain caused by imbalance in the muscles of the torso.

The format here is the same as that for the previous two major sections. Each section is presented as follows:

- Origin, insertion, and action of muscle(s), with illustration
- Detailed stretching instructions, with illustrations
- Alternative stretching instructions, where appropriate, with illustrations

QUADRATUS LUMBORUM

The quadratus lumborum (QL) is an important component of a strong and healthy low back. When this muscle is hypertonic, it develops trigger points that refer pain to the hips, gluteal area, and down the leg. The QL is always involved in low back pain, even that which results from disc problems or misalignment of the lumbar vertebrae.

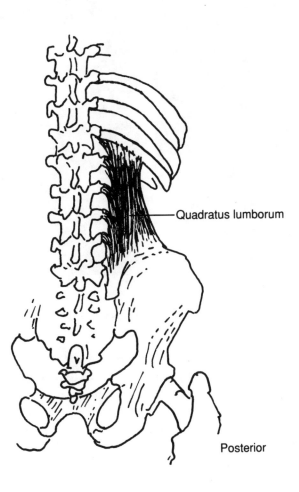

Quadratus lumborum

Posterior

Origin	Insertion	Action
Posterior iliac crest	Inferior border of the 12th rib and the transverse processes of L1-5	Lateral flexion of the trunk or elevation of the ilium

Instruction

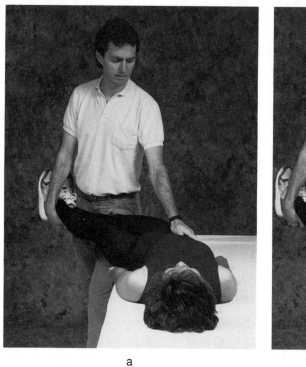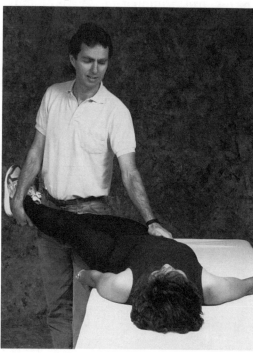

a   b

Figure 3.51   Initiation phase of the quadratus lumborum stretch: (a) Support the stretcher's legs; (b) assist while the stretcher deepens the stretch.

1. The stretcher lies supine, holding the sides of the table to prevent sliding off.

2. Grip both legs and pull them to one side, side-flexing the stretcher at the trunk as far as is comfortable for her. The stretcher keeps both hips flat on the table. This lengthens the QL to its pain-free end of range.

3. Stand between the table and the stretcher's legs, supporting them comfortably, and offer resistance to the isometric contraction of the QL (Figure 3.51a).

4. The stretcher attempts to elevate her ilium, isometrically contracting her QL, for 6 s. The stretcher begins slowly and builds to 50% to 100% of maximum, breathing throughout. Be certain that she is contracting the QL and not just pushing with her legs.

5. The stretcher relaxes, breathes deeply, and contracts the opposite QL to deepen the stretch (Figure 3.51b). You may *gently* push on the legs to assist the stretch.

6. Repeat 3 to 5 times.

Stretching should be pain-free. If the stretcher experiences pain during this stretch, try repositioning, or use less force during the isometric contraction. If pain persists, don't use PNF until you know the cause of the pain.

Alternative Instruction

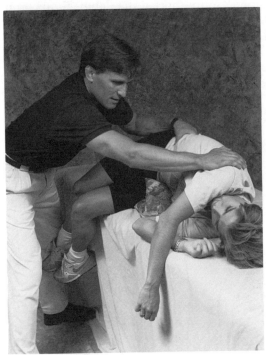 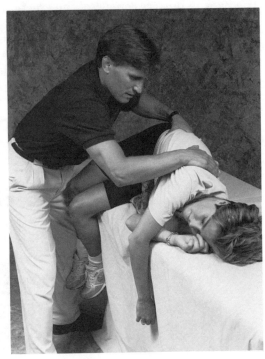

a   b

Figure 3.52   (a) Initiation phase of the alternate quadratus lumborum stretch. (b) Assist while the stretcher deepens the stretch.

1. The stretcher lies on her side, with her legs hanging off the side of the table. She has a pillow under her side, just above the iliac crest, to lengthen the QL to its pain-free end of range.

2. Position yourself facing the stretcher. Place one hand on her side between her iliac crest and her ribcage and your other hand on her shoulder. Place your leg against her feet to offer resistance to the isometric contraction of the QL (Figure 3.52a).

3. The stretcher pushes her feet and legs against you with enough force to engage the QL, isometrically contracting for 6 s. The stretcher begins slowly and builds to 50% to 100% of maximum, breathing throughout. Palpate with your hand to be certain she is contracting the QL and not just pushing with her legs.

4. The stretcher relaxes, breathes deeply, and pulls her legs away from you to deepen the stretch. *Gently* push on the legs to assist the stretch. You may also assist her to roll her shoulder forward to stretch the QL from the other end (Figure 3.52b).

5. Repeat 3 to 5 times.

Stretching should be pain-free. If the stretcher experiences pain during this stretch, try repositioning, or use less force during the isometric contraction. If pain persists, don't use PNF until you know the cause of the pain.

BACK EXTENSORS

The back extensors consist of the erector spinae group (iliocostalis, longissimus, and spinalis, each with two or three divisions) and the transversospinalis group (semispinalis, multifidus, rotatores, interspinalis, and intertransversarii). See Figure 3.53, a-c. We illustrate some of them here but are not listing the origins and insertions. These muscles, acting bilaterally, extend the spine. When they are hypertonic, they can create back pain and limit spinal flexion. They are also common sites for trigger points.

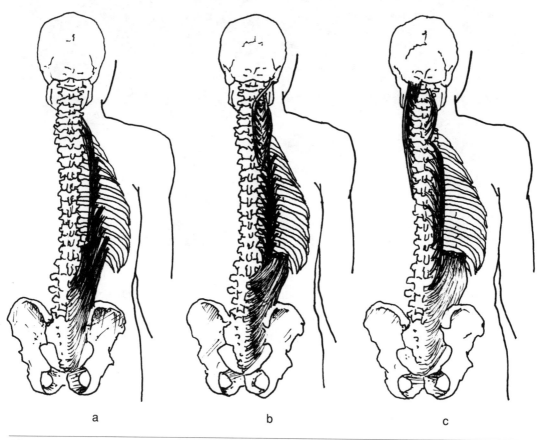

a   b   c

Figure 3.53   Erector spinae muscles: (a) iliocostalis, (b) longissimus, and (c) spinalis.

Instruction

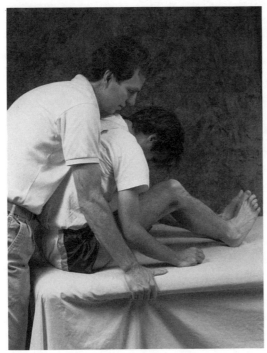
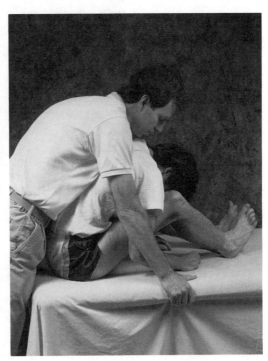

a   b

Figure 3.54   (a) Initiation phase for the back extensors stretch on the table. (b) The stretcher deepens the stretch.

1. The stretcher, seated at the edge of the treatment table with knees flexed, leans forward as far as possible by contracting the rectus abdominis and psoas. This lengthens the back extensors to their pain-free end of range.

2. Place your torso against the stretcher's back and hold the edges of the table to provide resistance to the isometric contraction of the back extensors (Figure 3.54a).

3. The stretcher attempts to extend his spine, isometrically contracting the back extensors, for 6 s. He does not use his arms to push back. The stretcher begins slowly and builds to 50% to 100% of maximum, breathing throughout.

4. The stretcher relaxes, breathes deeply, and contracts his rectus abdominis and psoas to deepen the stretch of the back extensors (Figure 3.54b). *Never push to deepen the stretch.*

5. Repeat 3 to 5 times, each time moving the resistance farther up the back. This stretch can also be done with the stretcher sitting on the floor. You offer resistance using your hands (Figure 3.55).

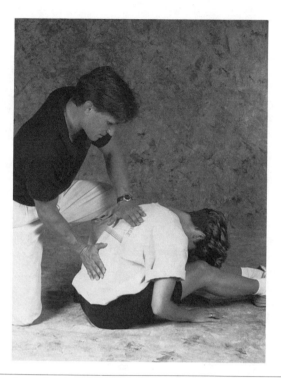

Figure 3.55   Initiation phase for the alternate back extensors stretch position on the floor.

Stretching should be pain-free. If the stretcher experiences pain during this stretch, try repositioning, or use less force during the isometric contraction. If pain persists, don't use PNF until you know the cause of the pain.

UPPER TRAPEZIUS

Many people have upper traps that are hypertonic. When the upper traps are too tight, they can cause headaches and pain. They also develop significant trigger points.

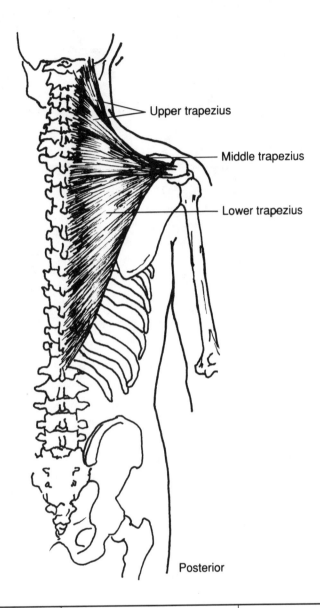

Origin	Insertion	Action
Occiput, spinous processes of C7-T12 and the ligamentum nuchae	Lateral clavicle, acromion	Elevation and upward rotation of the scapula

Instruction

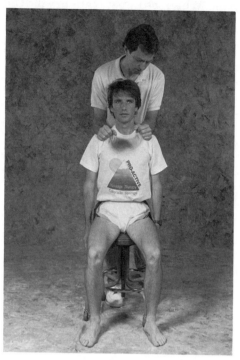
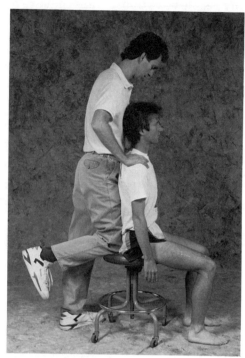

a   b

Figure 3.56   (a) Initiation position using a stool. (b) Use your leg to ensure the stretcher keeps a straight back.

1. The stretcher is seated on a low stool, with his back straight. He pulls his shoulders downward (depresses his scapulae), lengthening the upper traps to their pain-free end of range.

2. Place one forearm on each of the stretcher's shoulders to provide resistance to the isometric contraction of the upper trapezius (Figure 3.56a). Support the stretcher's back with your leg to prevent him from collapsing his spine (Figure 3.56b).

3. The stretcher attempts to shrug his shoulders, isometrically contracting the upper trapezii, for 6 s. He begins slowly and builds to 50% to 100% of maximum, breathing throughout.

4. The stretcher relaxes, breathes deeply, then pulls his shoulders downward, keeping the spine straight, to deepen the upper trapezii stretch. *Never push to deepen the stretch.*

5. Repeat 3 to 5 times.

Stretching should be pain-free. If the stretcher experiences pain during this stretch, try repositioning, or use less force during the isometric contraction. If pain persists, don't use PNF until you know the cause of the pain.

4

Using Spiral-
Diagonal Patterns

The single-muscle stretches covered in the last chapter are grounded in PNF principles but do not use the spiral-diagonal patterns of PNF. The heart of PNF is the spiral-diagonal movement patterns developed by Kabat, Knott, and Voss. These patterns closely resemble normal movements found in sports and physical activities and are called "mass movement patterns," defined by Voss et al. (1985) as "various combinations of motion . . . [that] require shortening and lengthening reactions of many muscles in varying degrees" (p. 1). The spiral-diagonal character of these normal movement patterns arises from the design of the skeletal system and the placement of the muscles on it. The muscles spiral around the bones from origin to insertion, and therefore, when they contract, they tend to create that spiral in motion (Figure 4.1, a-c).

Imagine a robot, whose arms and legs move in only one or two planes, stiff and awkward. Now take a walk around the room and notice the fluidity of your own arm and leg motions. The difference between you and a robot is that your motions have a spiral-diagonal component. This is especially noticeable in the movements of your arms, which swing across your body as you walk or run. Most muscles are actually capable of motion in three planes.

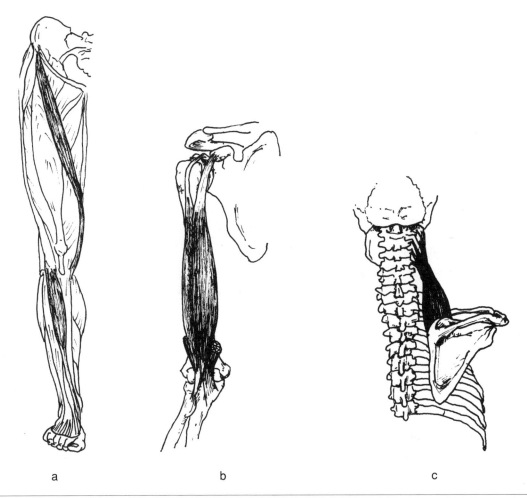

a   b   c

Figure 4.1   The attachments of (a) the sartorius and anterior tibialis, (b) the biceps brachii, and (c) the levator scapula muscles facilitate spiral-diagonal motion when the muscles contract.

For instance, the psoas muscle flexes the hip (the dominant action) but also assists adduction and external rotation of the femur (Figure 4.2). The spiral-diagonal patterns of PNF activate the muscles in all three planes of motion.

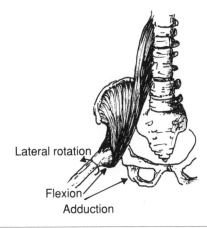

Figure 4.2   Many muscles, like the iliopsoas, create motion through three planes of movement.

The objectives for this chapter are to

- explain the spiral-diagonal patterns and how they differ from the single-muscle stretches,
- demonstrate the CRAC technique using the spiral diagonals,
- teach how to practice the patterns as free-movement exercises, enabling you to learn them kinesthetically as well as visually,
- provide detailed instruction, with illustrations, of the CRAC sequences for the upper and lower extremities, and
- discuss the additional complexities and benefits that arise from using the spiral-diagonal patterns.

Applying Spiral-Diagonal Patterns to CRAC Stretching

The full spiral-diagonal patterns use movement through three planes of motion: extension or flexion, adduction or abduction, and rotation. (Refer to the glossary for definitions of these terms.) When a physical therapist uses these PNF patterns, she or he uses movement through the full pattern to restore or increase strength and coordination, as well as to increase range of motion.

Because we are working with well-conditioned, uninjured people, our primary goal is to increase their range of motion quickly and efficiently. Using these three-dimensional PNF patterns, we stretch groups of related muscles simultaneously, thereby gaining greater benefit in a shorter amount of time, compared to the single-muscle stretches.

For stretching, we employ only the lengthened position of the pattern, without allowing the limb to go through its complete range of motion. The stretcher assumes the lengthened range (initiation phase) of the pattern, but during the contraction phase, you allow motion only in the rotational direction. The other two components of motion are resisted isometrically. According to Voss et al. (1985), rotation is what activates the muscles during a pattern, so rotation should be allowed while the other motions are resisted. We allow rotation to occur because it allows a stronger contraction in the other two planes.

Learning the Patterns

Voss et al. (1985) suggest learning the PNF patterns through free-movement exercises. These give a sense of the natural rhythm of the patterns and let you feel the movements through a full range of motion. The patterns are named for their ending positions. You may find this confusing at first, because you begin in the position that is opposite from the named diagonal. Learning the full pattern will make it easier to visualize the range of motion you are trying to improve and to understand the method of naming.

Patterns for the Arm

There are two basic PNF patterns for the arm: D1 and D2. Each pattern is divided into two parts: flexion and extension. You can see by studying Figure 4.3, a-c, that the movement sequence for the D1 extension pattern is the exact opposite of the sequence for D1 flexion (Figure 4.3, c-a). The same is true for D2 flexion and D2 extension.

D1 Patterns

The first pattern is called D1 (*D* is for diagonal) and is divided into D1 flexion (flexion-adduction–external rotation) and D1 extension (extension-abduction–internal rotation). Take a moment and practice these two patterns before going on. Stand up and place your right shoulder in full flexion, horizontal adduction, and external rotation. The right forearm is in supination, the wrist and fingers are flexed. Go as far in each plane of motion as you can to fully lengthen all the involved muscles. This is the

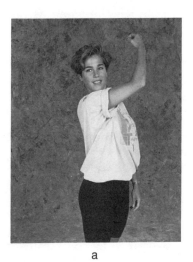
a

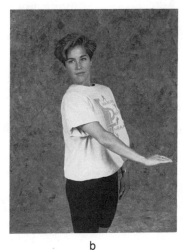
b

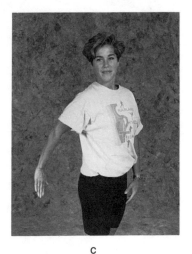
c

Figure 4.3 Free movements demonstrating PNF patterns for the upper extremity. D1 extension (swimmer's stretch): (a) initiation, (b) midphase, and (c) end position. D1 flexion (self-feed): (c) initiation, (b) midphase, and (a) end position.

initiation phase of D1 extension. You should be in the same position as the model in Figure 4.3a. Now, slowly move your arm diagonally, beginning with internal rotation at the wrist, into full extension, abduction, and internal rotation. The forearm pronates, wrist and fingers extend. This brings you to the end position of D1 extension, which is also the starting position of D1 flexion. You should be in the same position as the model in Figure 4.3c. The D1 flexion pattern begins where D1 extension terminates and simply retraces the previous motion. Repeat these patterns several times with each arm, and then with both together, until you feel the rhythm. What activities use motion like this? Throwing a frisbee, swinging a golf club or a baseball bat, picking up a hat and putting it on your head, working as a grocery checker: These all use patterns of mass movement that have components of the D1 pattern. The D1 flexion pattern can be thought of as the "self-feeding" pattern. The D1 extension pattern is sometimes referred to as the "swimmers' stretch." Figure 4.4 shows a pair of swimmers helping one another stretch before a meet. Notice the arm position of the swimmer being stretched.

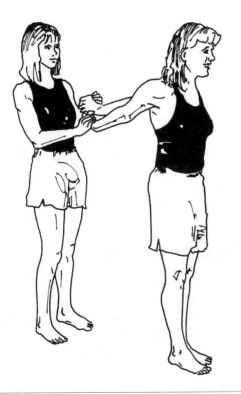

Figure 4.4   A pair of swimmers stretching. The arm position of the stretcher resembles the D1 extension pattern.

D2 Patterns

The second pattern, D2, uses the diagonal opposite to D1. D2 is also divided into two sections: D2 flexion (flexion-abduction–external rotation) and D2 extension (extension-adduction–internal rotation). Once again, practice these patterns now. Stand up and place your shoulder in full flexion, abduction, and external rotation. The forearm is supinated, the wrist and fingers extended. Remember, go as far into each plane of motion as possible. Check your position against the model in Figure 4.5a. This is the starting position of D2 extension. Now, slowly move your arm diagonally, beginning with rotation at the wrist, into extension, adduction, and internal rotation. The forearm is pronated, the wrist and fingers flexed. This is the end of D2 extension and the starting position of D2 flexion. Compare your position to Figure 4.5c. The D2 flexion pattern begins where D2 extension terminates, and simply retraces the previous motion. Practice these patterns until they feel comfortable and you sense their rhythm. What activities make use of these mass movement patterns of D2? Throwing a ball, drawing a sword, using a hockey stick, lifting and stacking, washing windows. To make it easier to remember the D2 flexion pattern, we'll call it "drawing a sword." You can remember the D2 extension pattern as "sheathing a sword."

CRAC Sequence for the Arms

CRAC stretching using the spiral-diagonal patterns is simple and straightforward. The sequence of steps is much the same as for the single-muscle stretches, except that we are using the starting position of a three-plane pattern. The D2 extension pattern (sheathing a sword) is the easiest to learn, so I'll use that as an example (see Figure 4.5a):

1. The stretcher, supine on the table, fully flexes, abducts, and externally rotates her shoulder. The forearm is supinated, the wrist and fingers extended. This is the starting position of D2 extension and lengthens the muscles we are about to stretch: pectorals, anterior deltoid, subscapularis, latissimus dorsi, pronator teres, and wrist and finger flexors.

2. Provide resistance as the stretcher attempts to initiate the pattern, beginning with internal rotation at the wrist. Maximally resist but allow rotation (isotonic contraction) at the wrist and arm and prevent adduction or exten-

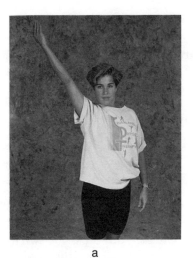 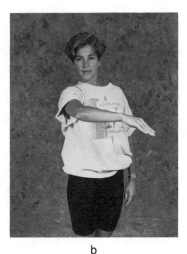 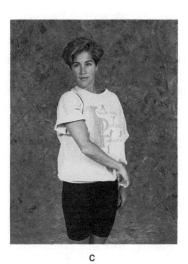

a b c

Figure 4.5 Free movements demonstrating the PNF patterns for the upper extremity. D2 extension (sheath sword): (a) initiation, (b) midphase, and (c) end position. D2 flexion (draw sword): (c) initiation, (b) midphase, and (a) end position.

sion (isometric contraction) of the shoulder (Figure 4.6a).

3. The contractions build slowly to 50% to 100% of maximum, with the stretcher (and yourself!) breathing throughout. After 6 s of contraction, the stretcher relaxes and takes a deep breath while you support her arm.

4. The stretcher then actively moves her arm farther into the lengthened range of the D2 extension pattern (Figure 4.6b). Support the arm, but *do not push to deepen the stretch*.

Important Differences

One difference in using CRAC with the spiral-diagonal patterns, compared to single-muscle stretches, is that you maximally resist but allow rotation of the arm while preventing any movement in the other two planes of motion (flexion-extension or adduction-abduction). The resistance you offer is graded to match the stretcher's contraction. As the stretcher increases effort to 50% to 100% of maximum, you increase resistance. This ensures maximal recruitment of muscle fibers, while still allowing rotation and preventing any other movement. Another important difference occurs when the stretcher deepens the stretch (Figure 4.6b). She must move as fully as possible into the lengthened range of all three planes of the pattern, especially rotation, to maximize the stretch.

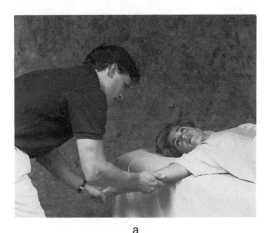 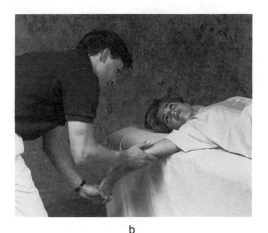

a b

Figure 4.6 Initiation phase of D2 extension: (a) The right arm is flexed, abducted, and externally rotated; (b) the stretcher actively deepens the stretch.

Patterns for the Leg

If you feel comfortable with your mastery of the arm patterns, it's time to move on to the legs. The patterns are very similar to those for the arms, but with enough variation to keep you on your toes. As with the arms, the leg patterns are called D1 and D2, and each has two parts. Remember, the patterns are named for their ending positions.

D1 Patterns

D1 is divided into D1 extension (extension-abduction–internal rotation, Figure 4.7, a-c) and D1 flexion (flexion-adduction–external rotation, Figure 4.7, c-a). Take some time before going on, and practice this pattern. Stand up and place your right leg into flexion, adduction, and external rotation. The foot is dorsiflexed and inverted, and the toes are extended. It may be helpful to use a chair or the wall for support. Compare your position to Figure 4.7a. This is the starting position for D1 extension. Slowly swing your leg, beginning with internal rotation. The foot and ankle plantarflex and evert, and the toes flex as the leg moves into abduction and extension, as in Figure 4.7c. This is the end of D1 extension and the beginning position of D1 flexion. The D1 flexion pattern begins where D1 extension terminates, and simply retraces the previous motion. Swing your leg through this pattern several times. Does it feel natural? D1 flexion is sometimes re-

ferred to as the "soccer kick." You can remember D1 extension as "toe-off." What activities require aspects of the whole D1 pattern? Dancers, soccer players, and skaters all use it.

D2 Patterns

D2 consists of D2 flexion (flexion-abduction–internal rotation) and D2 extension (extension-adduction–external rotation). To practice this pattern, stand up and place your leg in flexion, abduction, and internal rotation. The foot is dorsiflexed and everted, and the toes are extended. Check your position with the model in Figure 4.8a. Does this feel awkward? This is the initiation phase of D2 extension. Slowly swing your leg back, beginning with external rotation. The foot and ankle plantarflex and invert, and the toes flex as the leg moves into extension and adduction. This is the end of D2 extension and, naturally, the beginning of D2 flexion. You should be in the same position as the model in Figure 4.8c. The D2 flexion pattern begins where D2 extension terminates, and simply retraces the previous motion. Practice this a few times, until it begins to feel more natural. Does it remind you of anything? If you're a skier, you may recognize components of the snowplow turn in the D2 flexion pattern. To help you remember D2 flexion, we'll call it the "snowplow." The D2 extension pattern reminds some people of a ballet position, so we'll call it "turnout."

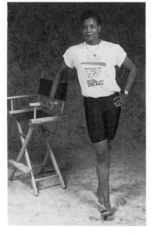
a

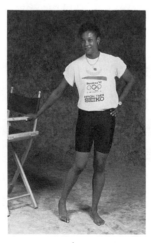
b

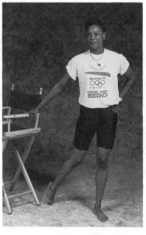
c

Figure 4.7   Free movements demonstrating PNF patterns for the lower extremity. D1 extension (toe-off): (a) initiation, (b) midphase, and (c) end position. D1 flexion (soccer kick): (c) initiation, (b) midphase, and (a) end position.

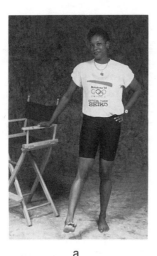
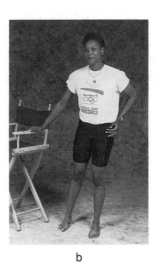
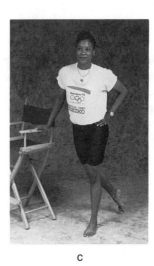

a   b   c

Figure 4.8   Free movements demonstrating PNF patterns for the lower extremity. D2 extension (turnout): (a) initiation, (b) midphase, and (c) end position. D2 flexion (snow plow): (c) initiation, (b) midphase, and (a) end position.

CRAC Sequence for the Legs

Now it's time to practice a CRAC stretch for the leg. We'll use the D1 extension pattern (toe-off) because it's the easiest to do.

1. The stretcher lies supine on the table. He raises his leg into flexion, adduction, and external rotation. The foot is dorsiflexed and in-verted, and the toes are extended. This is the initiation phase of D1 extension. This length-ens the muscles to be stretched: hamstrings (especially biceps femoris), gluteals, TFL, gas-trocnemius (lateral head), peroneals.

2. Support the leg and offer resistance to the stretcher's effort (Figure 4.9a). Allow inter-nal rotation, but not abduction or extension.

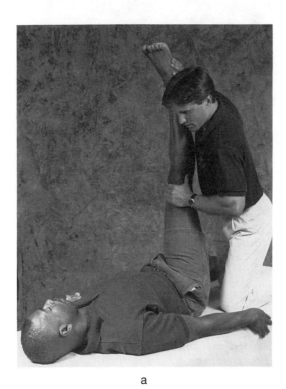
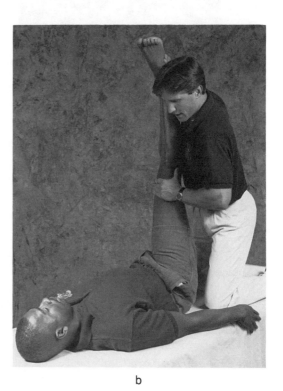

a   b

Figure 4.9   Initiation phase of D1 extension: (a) Stretcher's right leg is flexed, adducted, and externally rotated; (b) the stretcher actively deepens the stretch.

3. The stretcher attempts, for 6 s, to initiate the pattern (extension, abduction, and internal rotation), beginning with rotation and building slowly to 50% to 100% of maximum, breathing throughout.

4. The stretcher relaxes, takes a deep breath, and actively deepens the stretch by pulling his leg farther into flexion, adduction, and, especially, external rotation (Figure 4.9b). Support the leg, but *do not assist in deepening the stretch*.

Important Differences

Once again, the primary differences from the single-muscle stretches are related to the three-dimensional character of the patterns. Maximally resist, but allow rotation to occur, and prevent abduction or extension. When the stretcher deepens the stretch, he must go fully into all three planes of motion to maximize the benefits of PNF.

STRETCHES FOR THE UPPER EXTREMITIES

Now that you have a basic understanding of the spiral-diagonal patterns and how to apply them to CRAC stretching, we can go into more detail as we present the various stretches for the arms.

D1 EXTENSION (SWIMMER'S STRETCH)

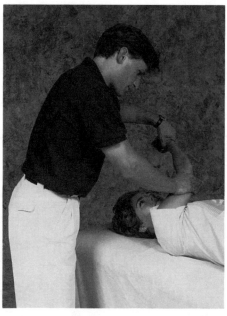
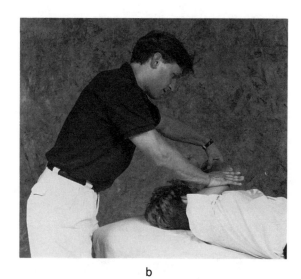

a   b

Figure 4.10 Initiation phase of D1 extension: (a) Stretcher's right shoulder is flexed, adducted, and externally rotated. The forearm is supinated, with wrist and fingers flexed. (b) The stretcher moves farther into flexion, adduction, and external rotation.

1. The stretcher lies supine, with the right shoulder flexed, adducted, and externally rotated. It may be helpful here to think of grabbing the ear on the opposite side. The forearm is supinated and the wrist and fingers flexed. This position lengthens the target muscles to their end range. These include the infraspinatus, middle trapezius, rhomboids, teres minor, posterior deltoid, and pronator teres.

2. Support and stabilize the arm (Figure 4.10a). Resist, but allow internal rotation, and prevent abduction and extension.

3. The stretcher attempts, for 6 s, to initiate the D1 extension pattern, beginning with internal rotation, then abduction, then extension. The stretcher begins slowly and builds to 50% to 100% of maximum contraction, breathing throughout.

4. The stretcher relaxes, takes a deep breath, and moves farther into flexion, adduction, and external rotation (Figure 4.10b). Support the arm, but *do not push to deepen the stretch*.

5. Repeat 3 to 5 times.

Stretching should be pain-free. If the stretcher experiences pain during this stretch, try repositioning the arm, or use less force during the resisted contraction phase. If pain persists, stop using PNF until you know the cause of the pain.

D1 FLEXION (SELF-FEEDING)

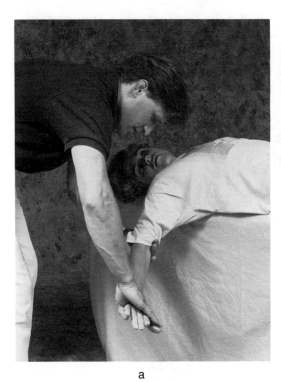
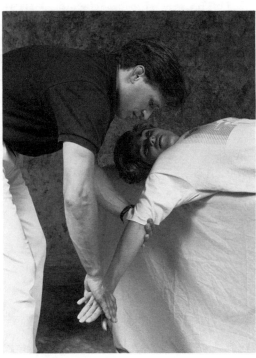

a   b

Figure 4.11   Initiation phase of D1 flexion: (a) Stretcher's right shoulder is fully extended, abducted, and internally rotated. The forearm is pronated with the wrist and fingers extended. (b) The stretcher moves farther into extension, abduction, and internal rotation.

1. The stretcher lies supine, with the right shoulder fully extended, abducted, and internally rotated. The forearm is pronated, the wrist and fingers extended. This position lengthens the target muscles to their end range. These include the pectorals (clavicular head), anterior deltoid, coracobrachialis, biceps brachii, infraspinatus, and supinator.

2. Support and stabilize the arm (Figure 4.11a). Resist, but allow external rotation, and prevent adduction and flexion.

3. The stretcher attempts, for 6 s, to initiate the D1 flexion pattern, beginning with external rotation, then adduction, then flexion. She begins slowly and builds to 50% to 100% of maximum contraction, breathing throughout.

4. The stretcher relaxes, takes a deep breath, and moves farther into extension, abduction, and internal rotation (Figure 4.11b). Support the arm, but *do not push to deepen the stretch*.

5. Repeat 3 to 5 times.

Stretching should be pain-free. If the stretcher experiences pain during this stretch, try repositioning the arm, or use less force during the resisted contraction phase. If pain persists, stop using PNF until you know the cause of the pain.

D2 FLEXION (DRAWING A SWORD)

1. The stretcher lies prone, with the right shoulder extended, adducted, and internally rotated. The forearm is pronated, the wrist and fingers flexed. This position lengthens the target muscles to their end range. These include the anterior deltoid, coracobrachialis, pectorals, biceps brachii, and supinator.

2. Support and stabilize the arm (Figure 4.12). Resist, but allow external rotation, and prevent abduction and flexion.

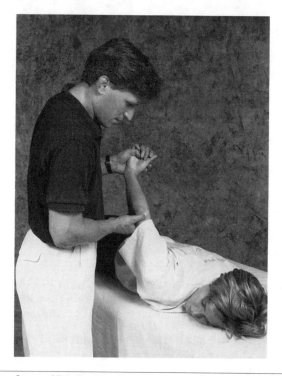

Figure 4.12   Initiation phase of D2 flexion: Stretcher's right shoulder is extended, adducted, and internally rotated. The forearm is pronated with the wrist and fingers flexed.

3. The stretcher attempts, for 6 s, to initiate the D2 flexion pattern, beginning with external rotation, then abduction, then flexion. She begins slowly and builds to 50% to 100% of maximum contraction, breathing throughout.

4. The stretcher relaxes, takes a deep breath, and moves farther into extension, adduction, and internal rotation. Support the arm, but *do not push to deepen the stretch*.

5. Repeat 3 to 5 times.

Stretching should be pain-free. If the stretcher experiences pain during this stretch, try repositioning the arm, or use less force during the resisted contraction phase. If pain persists, stop using PNF until you know the cause of the pain.

D2 EXTENSION (SHEATHING A SWORD)

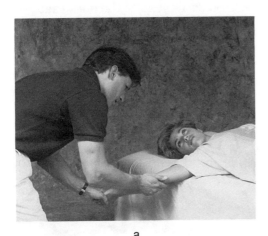
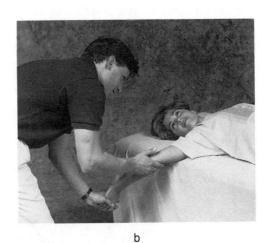

a   b

Figure 4.13 Initiation phase of D2 extension: (a) The stretcher's right shoulder is fully flexed, abducted, and externally rotated. The forearm is supinated with the wrist and fingers extended. (b) The stretcher moves farther into flexion, abduction, and external rotation.

1. The stretcher lies supine, with the right shoulder fully flexed, abducted, and externally rotated. The forearm is supinated, the wrist and fingers extended. This position lengthens the target muscles to their end range. These include the pectorals (sternal head), anterior deltoid, subscapularis, pronator teres, latissimus dorsi, and teres major.

2. Support and stabilize the arm (Figure 4.13a). Maximally resist, but allow internal rotation, and prevent adduction and extension.

3. The stretcher attempts, for 6 s, to initiate the D2 extension pattern, beginning with internal rotation at the wrist, then adduction, then extension. She begins slowly and builds to 50% to 100% of maximum contraction, breathing throughout.

4. The stretcher relaxes, takes a deep breath, and moves further into flexion, abduction, and external rotation (Figure 4.13b). Support the arm, but *do not push to deepen the stretch*.

5. Repeat 3 to 5 times.

Stretching should be pain-free. If the stretcher experiences pain during this stretch, try repositioning the arm, or use less force during the resisted contraction phase. If pain persists, stop using PNF until you know the cause of the pain.

STRETCHES FOR THE LOWER EXTREMITIES

Not all of the leg patterns lend themselves to CRAC stretching. For instance, the D2 flexion pattern is extremely awkward to carry out. So we'll practice the ones that are the easiest to learn and use. If you have special circumstances with a particular stretcher, be creative in developing other stretches based on PNF principles and the patterns for the leg.

D1 EXTENSION (TOE-OFF)

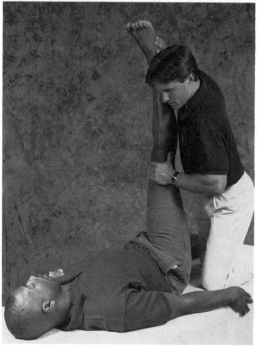 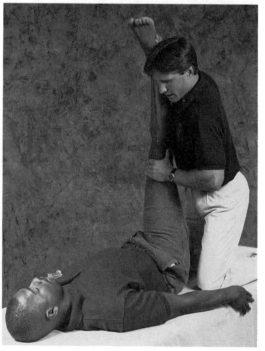

a   b

Figure 4.14   Initiation phase of D1 extension: (a) Stretcher's right leg is flexed, adducted, and externally rotated. The foot is dorsiflexed and inverted, and the toes are extended. (b) The stretcher moves the hip farther into flexion, adduction, and external rotation and increases dorsiflexion and inversion of the foot and extension of the toes.

1. The stretcher lies supine, with the right leg in flexion, adduction, and external rotation. The foot is dorsiflexed and inverted, and the toes are extended. This is the starting position for D1 extension and lengthens the target muscles to their end range. These include the hamstrings (especially biceps femoris), gluteals, TFL, gastrocnemius (especially lateral head), soleus, and peroneals.

2. Support and stabilize the leg (Figure 4.14a). Maximally resist, but allow rotation, and prevent abduction and extension.

3. The stretcher attempts, for 6 s, to initiate the D1 extension pattern, beginning with internal rotation, then abduction, then extension. He begins slowly and builds to 50% to 100% of maximum contraction, breathing throughout.

4. The stretcher relaxes, takes a deep breath, and moves the hip farther into flexion, adduction, and external rotation. He increases dorsiflexion and inversion of the foot and extension of the toes (Figure 4.14b). Support the leg, but *do not push to deepen the stretch*.

5. Repeat 3 to 5 times.

Stretching should be pain-free. If the stretcher experiences pain during this stretch, try repositioning the leg, or use less force during the resisted contraction phase. If pain persists, stop using PNF until you know the cause of the pain.

D1 FLEXION (SOCCER KICK)

Because the stretcher is prone in this stretch, you may be somewhat confused between internal and external rotation. Pay attention only to the thigh and ignore the position of the lower leg and foot when determining which is internal and which is external rotation.

1. The stretcher lies prone, with the right knee flexed and the hip in extension, abduction, and internal rotation. For this stretch, the position of the foot and toes is not important. The knee is in flexion here to make it easier for the stretcher to lift his leg off the table. This is the starting position of D1 flexion and lengthens the target muscles to their end range. These include the iliopsoas, the rectus femoris, the adductors, and the lateral hip rotators.

2. Support and stabilize the leg, at the same time stabilizing the hips to keep them on the table (Figure 4.15a). Maximally resist, but allow external rotation, and prevent adduction and flexion.

3. The stretcher attempts, for 6 s, to initiate the D1 flexion pattern, beginning with external rotation, then adduction, then flexion. He begins slowly and builds to 50% to 100% of maximum contraction, breathing throughout.

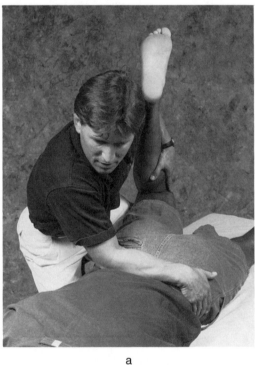 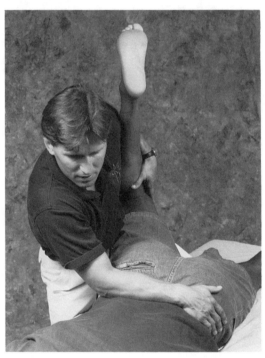

a   b

Figure 4.15   Initiation phase of D1 flexion: (a) Stretcher is prone with right knee flexed and with hip extended, abducted, and internally rotated. (b) Stretcher moves leg farther into extension, abduction, and internal rotation. Hold the stretcher's hips to the table.

4. The stretcher relaxes, takes a deep breath, and moves his leg farther into extension, abduction, and internal rotation (Figure 4.15b). You must stabilize the pelvis here to keep both hips on the table. Support the leg, but *do not assist to deepen the stretch*.

5. Repeat 3 to 5 times.

> **Stretching should be pain-free. If the stretcher experiences pain during this stretch, try repositioning the leg, or use less force during the resisted contraction phase. If pain persists, stop using PNF until you know the cause of the pain.**

D2 EXTENSION (TURNOUT)

1. The stretcher lies supine, with the right leg flexed, abducted, and internally rotated. The foot is dorsiflexed and everted, and the toes are extended. This is the starting position for D2 extension and lengthens the target muscles to their end range. These include the gluteals, hamstrings (medial), gastrocnemius (especially medial head), soleus, gracilis, adductors, and posterior tibialis.

2. Support and stabilize the leg (Figure 4.16a). Maximally resist, but allow external rotation, and prevent adduction and extension.

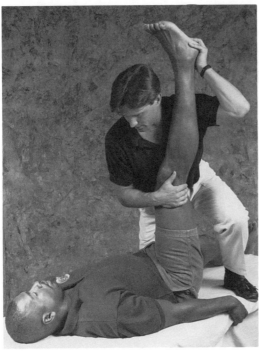
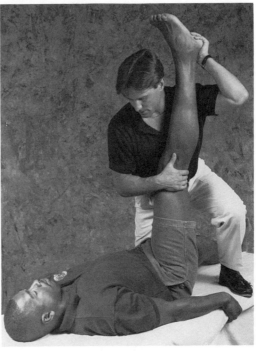

a   b

Figure 4.16 Initiation phase of D2 extension: (a) Stretcher's right hip is flexed, abducted, and internally rotated. The foot is dorsiflexed and everted, and the toes are extended. (b) The stretcher moves hip farther into flexion, abduction, and internal rotation and increases dorsiflexion and eversion of the foot and extension of the toes.

3. The stretcher attempts, for 6 s, to initiate the D2 extension pattern, beginning with external rotation, then adduction, then extension. He begins slowly and builds to 50% to 100% of maximum contraction, breathing throughout.

4. The stretcher relaxes, takes a deep breath, and moves the hip farther into flexion, abduction, and internal rotation. He increases dorsiflexion and eversion of the foot and extension of the toes (Figure 4.16b). Support the leg, but *do not push to deepen the stretch*.

5. Repeat 3 to 5 times.

Stretching should be pain-free. If the stretcher experiences pain during this stretch, try repositioning the leg or using less force during the resisted contraction phase. If pain persists, stop using PNF until you know the cause of the pain.

5

Rehabilitation and PNF

Jeff Charland, RPT, ATC

Rehabilitation involves much more than simply regaining range of motion—it must also address strength, speed, endurance, and normal function. In this chapter I'll describe how various PNF techniques are employed in the rehabilitation of injuries. You'll see that PNF is a multilayered modality that is useful in every stage of rehabilitation.

The primary focus of this book is an "unimpaired" population. What has been presented so far is one PNF technique (CRAC stretching) of the many that are used by skilled practitioners. Though this chapter can't give you a complete working knowledge of PNF as it is employed during rehabilitation, you'll get an informative overview.

In this chapter we'll

- discuss the goals of rehabilitation;
- provide examples of the variety of conditions that benefit from PNF;
- discuss modalities used in rehabilitating sport injuries; and
- examine a specific rehabilitation scenario for an in-depth look at the way a program is developed to restore flexibility, strength, endurance, and speed.

Goals of Rehabilitation

The goal of a rehabilitation program is to restore an injured area to preinjury status or better. Results are charted by comparing pain level, strength, range of motion, and function before and after injury. These factors are monitored closely to ensure progress, and the initial rehabilitation program is altered as necessary during the course of treatment to keep the patient on track with the healing process.

During rehabilitation, a full range of PNF techniques may be used to stretch and strengthen muscles in a functional, coordinated manner. The specific techniques include approximation, traction, hold-relax active motion (similar to CRAC), rhythmic initiation, rhythmic stabilization, rhythmic rotation, slow reversal, slow reversal hold, quick reversal, contract-relax, and hold-relax. (For further information about these techniques, consult Voss et al., 1985).

The Many Uses for PNF

A wide array of conditions lend themselves to PNF techniques. For example, a person who sustains a severe head injury or a stroke resulting in central nervous system damage (to the brain or spinal cord) will require extensive rehabilitation to retrain damaged neuromuscular pathways. PNF is perhaps the most valuable tool for restoring normal movement patterns, strength, endurance, and, ultimately, full function. Rehabilitation of a back injury requires segmental and multisegmental stabilization techniques, which are found in the PNF repertoire. Following immobilization of a fracture, full range of motion, strength, and function need to be restored in the affected body segment. PNF can be invaluable to achieve this goal.

A baseball pitcher with a torn rotator cuff will require aggressive PNF strengthening and stretching following surgery to be able to return to throwing. A therapist can use PNF stretching to help a burn patient improve joint range of motion by mobilizing scars and stretching skin grafts. These examples illustrate but a few of the ways PNF can be incorporated into a rehabilitation program.

General Guidelines for Rehabilitation

Now that you have a better appreciation for the role of PNF in rehabilitation, I'll discuss the general guidelines for rehabilitating an overuse sport injury. Whatever your sport—tennis, running, biking, swimming, hiking, and so on—you've probably experienced pain due to overuse. Whenever you increase the intensity or duration of exercise, you run the risk of soft-tissue injury, which results in inflammation.

Inflammation

Inflammation is your body's normal response to injury, but it must be controlled. Histamine released into the injured area causes blood vessels to dilate, bringing more nutrients to the injury site to help heal the tissues but also causing swelling. Pain results from pressure on the free nerve endings in the swollen area. (Swelling can also result from bleeding from larger vessels or trauma to ligaments or bone. Our discussion is focused on microvascular damage due to minor overuse injuries.) Swelling also interferes with healing by reducing the oxygen supply to the injured tissue. Minor overuse injuries usually heal by themselves with proper rest and perhaps the use of ice and nonsteroidal anti-inflammatory medication. Problems arise when we ignore these mild symptoms and continue to train or perform the activity that caused the initial response.

A physical therapist or certified athletic trainer usually sees patients with inflammation after they've seen a doctor for pain or injury that "just won't go away" or is getting worse. The initial goals in therapy are to reduce the inflammation (which will reduce the pain) and concomitantly restore passive range of motion.

There are a number of ways to reduce inflammation. Cold is the most widely used modality to control inflammation and swelling, reduce muscle spasm, and relieve pain. It's typically applied using ice packs or ice massage.

Several electrical modalities can be helpful, such as electrical stimulation (AC-alternating current, low frequency, high frequency, surged, and varying wave forms), iontophoresis (delivery of medication via direct current), phonophoresis (delivery of medication via ultrasound), MENS (microcurrent), and many more "magic boxes" of all shapes and sizes.

Gentle passive range-of-motion exercise helps reduce joint pain and swelling. Isometric exercise helps pump away by-products and metabolites via the one-way valve system in the venous and lymphatic systems.

Scar Tissue

Once inflammation is reduced, scar tissue formation, weakness, and joint restrictions must be addressed. Scar tissue forms to replace normal tissue that's been injured. If the area is rested appropriately, scar tissue is minimized. But once it is formed, we must make the best of it. Normal collagen (tendons and ligaments are made of this) is a very tight, organized matrix with tremendous tensile strength. Scar tissue, on the other hand, is a disorganized, random array of collagen with a weaker tensile property. If the injury is not treated properly and promptly, this weaker tensile property contributes to reinjury. Deep transverse friction massage can move and stretch this scar tissue to make it more functional.

Joint Evaluation

Next, joint mechanics, namely, osteokinematics (range of motion) and arthrokinematics (sliding, gliding, and rolling of joint surfaces) are evaluated and restored if restrictions are present.

Heat

When acute inflammation has subsided, heat (deep or superficial) is often used to enhance blood flow to the area, resulting in increased elastic properties of the soft tissues for more effective stretching. Ultrasound and diathermy are deep forms of heat. Moist heat packs, warm whirlpool, and paraffin wax provide superficial heat. Once the tissue has been heated, PNF techniques can be used to effectively lengthen it without pain. This accomplishes two of the goals of rehabilitation: reduce pain and restore normal range of motion.

Muscle Strengthening

Once full joint mobility and soft-tissue flexibility (length) are achieved, our focus shifts to strengthening muscles. A strengthening program may include the use of isokinetic devices, weight machines, sport cords (surgical tubing is quite versatile), and free weights. PNF is perhaps the most efficient means of achieving strength gains in a specific area.

Most of the "machines" available fail to address one of the most important components of strengthening, namely, the rotational movements of a functional pattern. These machines, for the most part, strengthen only major muscle groups in one or two planes of motion and do not stress the stabilization of proximal (close to the torso) structures, which are crucial for proper function and maximal efficiency of the extremities. Several PNF techniques promote proximal stabilization (rhythmic stabilization and approximation, for example), whereas machines actually eliminate this important action when the person is strapped to the machine and the straps do all of this work.

Theoretical Case Study

As an example, let's take a baseball pitcher following arthroscopic decompression of the subacromial joint, a common procedure with rotator cuff injuries. Putting this athlete on a machine to build muscle strength will do very little for the scapulothoracic musculature. Free weights and machines can work the muscles only in one or two planes of motion, but the pitching motion occurs in a three-dimensional plane. There are many ways in which PNF allows us to accomplish the task of building strength, endurance, and power in a functional, three-dimensional manner. By utilizing the D2 extension pattern (Figure 5.1b), we can simulate the motion a pitcher uses while delivering a screwball. By reversing the rotation component of D2 extension (Figure 5.1c), we can simulate a curve ball. By resisting either D1 or D2 flexion patterns eccentrically, we are building the deceleration muscles, which are critical following release of the ball.

Muscles of Acceleration

The primary muscles that accelerate the arm in a pitch are the pectoralis major, latissimus dorsi, teres major, subscapularis, and triceps brachii. D1 and D2 extension patterns incorporate all but one of these, the triceps brachii. The triceps works only isometrically when we carry out the motion with the elbow extended. A nice

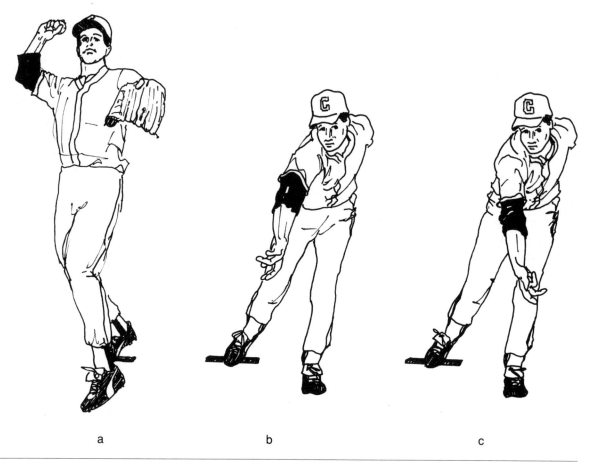

a   b   c

Figure 5.1   (a) When preparing to throw, this pitcher is in the starting position of the D2 extension pattern. (b) Pitching a screwball uses the normal D2 extension pattern. (c) Pitching a curveball reverses the usual rotation of D2 extension.

feature of PNF is that we can modify the techniques to include all the muscles that need work. Therefore, we can start either D1 or D2 extension with the elbow flexed to strengthen the triceps concentrically.

Muscles of Deceleration

The other major action of the pitching motion is deceleration after the ball is released. The primary muscles responsible for this are the biceps brachii, deltoid, supraspinatus, infraspinatus, teres minor, and scapular stabilizers (which will be discussed later). The biceps decelerates both the elbow and the glenohumeral joints. The supraspinatus, infraspinatus, and teres minor, in addition to dynamically stabilizing the glenohumeral joint during the cocking and acceleration phase, also decelerate the glenohumeral joint after release of the ball. Therefore, it is extremely important to strengthen these muscles, commonly referred to as the rotator

cuff, both concentrically and eccentrically. We do this by supplementing the PNF strengthening regimen with resistive exercises (e.g., free weights, surgical tubing) to build eccentric as well as concentric strength.

Muscles of Stabilization

When rehabilitating the throwing shoulder, we must also be aware of the importance of the scapular stabilizing muscles. The primary stabilizers (Figure 5.2) are the rhomboids, trapezius, levator scapula, and serratus anterior. From an anatomical and musculoskeletal standpoint, the arm is fairly useless without a strong base of support, which is provided by the scapula. If the muscles surrounding the scapula are weak, the muscles of the shoulder joint cannot work efficiently. The shoulder muscles not only are at a biomechanical disadvantage with weak scapular muscles, but also may be at higher risk of injury or reinjury. Therefore, it is imperative to include the scapular muscles during rehabilitation.

We can instruct the pitcher in several prone, sitting, or standing exercises that emphasize adduction of the scapula and horizontal abduction of the shoulder utilizing free weights, surgical tubing, or even some machines. Early on in the rehabilitation program, we can initiate scapular stabilization using rhythmic stabilization, rhythmic initiation, and approximation of the shoulder joint. All of these PNF techniques can achieve the desired outcome under the hands of a trained clinician.

PNF Stretching Patterns

Frequently, throwing athletes have strong, tight anterior (accelerating) muscles and relatively weak posterior muscles, creating significant muscle imbalance. PNF stretching can play an important role here. For example, to gain maximal elongation of the pectoralis major, we apply the CRAC technique at the beginning of D2 extension (Figure 5.3a). If the posterior

glenohumeral joint capsule is tight, we apply the CRAC technique at the beginning position of D1 extension (Figure 5.3b).

A Typical PNF Rehabilitation Session

Although each injured person has specific rehabilitation needs, there are certain commonalities. Certain modalities are used only in particular phases of rehabilitation; others are used throughout treatment. The following discussion, by no means a thorough look at the possible treatment programs that might be designed for the same injury, is offered as the outline of a program.

Warm-Up

Once the acute inflammation of an injury has subsided, a typical session may begin by first warming the joint and muscles by applying a moist heat pack for 20 min; or ultrasound for 5 to 10 min; or some light exercise for 10 min,

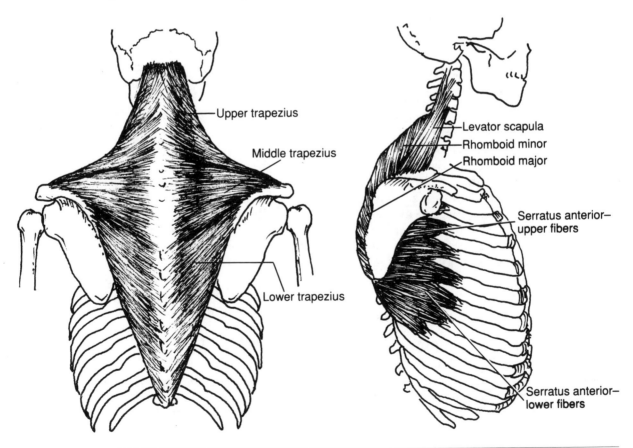

Figure 5.2 Scapular stabilizers: rhomboids, trapezius, levator scapula, and serratus anterior.

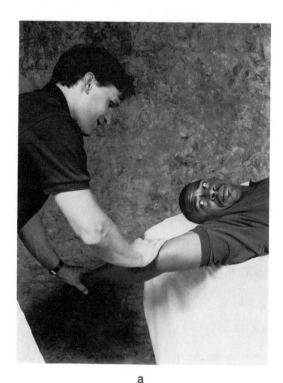
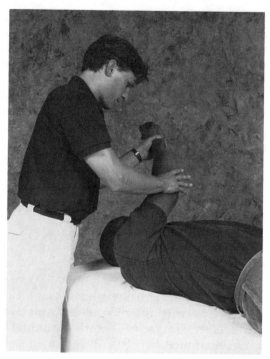

a   b

Figure 5.3   (a) Stretching the pectoralis major using the D2 extension pattern. (b) Stretching the posterior shoulder using the D1 extension pattern.

using pulleys, the upper body ergometer (UBE), or the stationary bike.

Preliminary Mobilization

Once the area is sufficiently warmed up, we can begin stretching. When treating a shoulder injury, we prefer to first have the patient use a T-bar (PVC shaped as a *T*) with an independent self-stretching routine. Next, we employ joint mobilization techniques to improve joint arthrokinematics so that PNF stretching will be more effective and comfortable. Once the muscles have adequate blood profusion (are warmed up) and the joint is mobile, we are ready to begin PNF stretching and strengthening.

PNF Stretching and Strengthening

We prefer to alternate sets of PNF stretching and strengthening. Depending on the athlete's fitness level and what we are trying to emphasize (strength, power, endurance), we may complete several sets of 10, 20, 30, or more repetitions of several patterns. Which patterns we use depend on our assessment as to which muscles are weaker, tighter, and so on.

Cryotherapy

Most clinicians prefer to ice the injured area following the session, in case the rehabilitation program causes inflammation. Ice can be applied via ice massage directly to the area for 5 to 10 min or an ice bag for no more than 20 to 30 min.

Conditioning

We include cardiovascular conditioning and general strengthening of the entire body in rehabilitation because the body heals faster if it's in good shape. People tend to be deconditioned after an injury because they've become inactive. Cardiovascular conditioning is usually done using a stationary bicycle, stairclimber, treadmill, UBE, or swimming pool. A weight training program is used to build or maintain overall strength, keeping in mind any restrictions related to the injured area.

Sport-Specific Training

Finally, once a good functional strength base is achieved and the patient has full range of motion without pain, we progress to the activity itself, utilizing sport-specific training. In the case of the baseball pitcher, we're now ready to initiate an interval throwing program or throwing a football (this slows down the throwing motion velocity). A runner, cyclist, or tennis player would use a similar progressive interval program to gradually return to full activity. A maintenance program is necessary to prevent reinjury and can usually be effective when done three times a week in conjunction with a normal training program.

Glossary

Abduction—Moving a limb away from the midline of the body, as in raising the arm horizontally

Adduction—Moving a limb toward the midline of the body, as in lowering the raised arm from the horizontal position

Dorsiflexion—Bending the foot upward

Eversion—Turning the foot so the sole faces outward

Extension—Movement at a joint so that the joint angle is increased and the parts move farther apart, as in straightening the elbow

Flexion—Movement at a joint so that the joint angle is decreased and the parts come closer together, as in bending the elbow

Horizontal abduction—Movement of the arm away from the midline of the body, beginning with the arm at shoulder level, as in using the right arm to draw a curtain from left to right

Horizontal adduction—Movement of the arm toward the midline of the body, beginning with the arm at shoulder level, as in using the right arm to open a curtain from right to left

Hyperextension—Movement of a joint beyond its normal position of extension, as in locking the knees back when standing

Inversion—Turning the foot so the sole faces inward

Plantarflexion—Bending the foot downward

Pronation—Turning the hand so the palm faces downward, as in palming a basketball

Rotation—The movement of a bone around an axis

Supination—Turning the hand so the palm faces upward, as in holding a bowl of soup

References

Anderson, B. (1984). *Stretching*. Bolinas, CA: Shelter.

Beaulieu, J.E. (1981). Developing a stretching program. *Physician and Sports Medicine*, **9**(11), 59-69.

Condon, S.M., & Hutton, R.S. (1987). Soleus muscle electromyographic activity and ankle dorsiflexion range of motion during four stretching procedures. *Physical Therapy*, **67**, 24-30.

Cornelius, W.L. (1983). Stretch evoked EMG activity by isometric contraction and submaximal concentric contraction. *Athletic Training*, **18**, 106-109.

Cornelius, W.L., & Craft-Hamm, K. (1988). Proprioceptive neuromuscular facilitation flexibility techniques: Acute effects on arterial blood pressure. *Physician and Sports Medicine*, **16**(4), 152-161.

Etnyre, B.R., & Abraham, L.D. (1986). Gains in range of ankle dorsiflexion using three popular stretching techniques. *American Journal of Physical Medicine*, **65**, 189-196.

Holt, L.E. (1976). *Scientific stretching for sport (3-S)*. Halifax, NS: Sport Research.

Lucas, R.C., & Koslow, R. (1984). Comparative study of static, dynamic, and proprioceptive neuromuscular facilitation stretching techniques on flexibility. *Perceptual Motor Skills*, **58**, 615-618.

Medeiros, J.M., Smidt, G.L., Burmeister, L.F., & Soderberg, G.L. (1977). The influence of isometric exercise and passive stretch on hip joint motion. *Physical Therapy*, **57**, 518-523.

Moore, M.A., & Hutton, R.S. (1980). Electromyographic investigation of muscle stretching techniques. *Medicine and Science in Sports and Exercise*, **12**, 322-329.

Osternig, L.R., Robertson, R., Troxel, R., & Hansen, P. (1987). Muscle activation during proprioceptive neuromuscular facilitation (PNF) stretching techniques. *American Journal of Physical Medicine*, **66**, 298-307.

Osternig, L.R., Robertson, R.N., Troxel, R.K., & Hansen, P. (1990). Differential responses to proprioceptive neuromuscular facilitation (PNF) stretch techniques. *Medicine and Science in Sports and Exercise*, **22**, 106-111.

Prentice, W.E. (1983). A comparison of static stretching and PNF stretching for improving hip joint flexibility. *Athletic Training*, **18**, 56-59.

Sady, S.P., Wortman, M., & Blanke, D. (1982). Flexibility training: Ballistic, static, or proprioceptive neuromuscular facilitation? *Archives of Physical Medicine and Rehabilitation*, **63**, 261-263.

Sapega, A.A., Quedenfeld, T.C., Moyer, R.A., & Butler, R.A. (1981). Biophysical factors in range-of-motion exercise. *Physician and Sports Medicine*, **9**(12), 57-65.

Surburg, P.R. (1981). Neuromuscular facilitation techniques in sportsmedicine. *Physician and Sports Medicine*, **9**(9), 115-127.

Surburg, P.R. (1983). Flexibility exercise re-examined. *Athletic Training*, **18**, 37-40.

Tanigawa, M.C. (1972). Comparison of the hold-relax procedure and passive mobilization on increasing muscle length. *Physical Therapy*, **52**, 725-735.

Taylor, D.C., Dalton, J.D., Seaber, A.V., & Garrett, W.E. (1990). Viscoelastic properties of muscle-tendon units: The biomechanical effects of stretching. *American Journal of Sports Medicine*, **18**, 300-309.

Voss, D., Ionta, M.K., & Myers, B. (1985). *Proprioceptive neuromuscular facilitation* (3rd ed.). Philadelphia: Harper & Row.

Index

A

Abraham, L.D., 12
Acceleration muscles, in rehabilitation, 95-96
Adductors, 38-42
    cautions for stretching, 39
    diagram and description of, 38-39
    functional assessment of, 39
    long adductor stretches, 38-39, 41
    partner stretches for, 40-41
    self-stretches for, 42
    short adductor stretches, 38, 40
Anderson, Bob, 5
Arms. *See* Upper extremity stretches, single-muscle; Upper
    extremity stretches, spiral-diagonal

B

Back extensors
    diagram and description of, 72
    partner stretches for, 73-74
Back pain, and psoas stretches, 29
Ballistic stretching
    description of, 6
    research on effectiveness of, 11
    risks with, 6
Beaulieu, J.E., 6, 10
Benefits of PNF stretches
    for injury prevention, 63
    for lower extremity flexibility, 16
    for massage, reducing discomfort of, 13
    for pain prevention/relief, 49, 68
    research on, 11
    of single-muscle stretches, 16
    of torso stretches, 68
    of wrist stretches, 60
Blanke, D., 11
Blood pressure increase with PNF, 10-11
Boston University, 2
Burmeister, L.F., 10
Butler, R.A., 11

C

Cardiovascular complications with PNF, 10-11
Cautions
    for adductor stretches, 39
    for iliacus stretches, 29
    for IT band stretches, 44
    for piriformis stretches, 49
    for psoas major stretches, 29
    for tensor fascia latae stretches, 44
    for wrist stretches, 63
Coghill, George, 9
Conditioning for rehabilitation, 98
Condon, S.M., 10
Contractions. *See* Muscle contractions
Contract-relax (CR). *See* CR (contract-relax)
Contract-relax, antagonist-contract (CRAC). *See* CRAC
    (contract-relax, antagonist-contract)
Cornelius, W.L., 10-11
CR (contract-relax)
    description of, 7
    research on effectiveness of, 12
CRAC (contract-relax, antagonist-contract)
    benefits of, 14
    description of, 8
    for rehabilitation, 97
    research on effectiveness of, 11-12
    for single-muscle stretches, 14-15
    for spiral-diagonal stretches, 78-84
Craft-Hamm, K., 11
Cryotherapy for rehabilitation, 98

D

D1 extension of arm (swimmer's stretch)
    instructions for stretch, 84-85
    movement patterns for, 79-80
    in rehabilitation, 95-96, 97
D1 extension of leg (toe-off)
    instructions for stretch, 88-89
    movement patterns for, 82, 83-84
D1 flexion of arm (self-feeding)
    instructions for stretch, 85-86
    movement patterns for, 79-80
    in rehabilitation, 95
D1 flexion of leg (soccer kick)
    instructions for stretch, 90-91
    movement patterns for, 82

D2 extension of arm (sheathing a sword)
  instructions for stretch, 87-88
  movement patterns for, 80-81
  in rehabilitation, 95-96, 97
D2 extension of leg (turnout)
  instructions for stretch, 91-92
  movement patterns for, 82
D2 flexion of arm (drawing a sword)
  instructions for stretch, 86-87
  movement patterns for, 80-81
  in rehabilitation, 95
D2 flexion of leg (snowplow), movement patterns for, 82
Dalton, J.D., 11
Deceleration muscles, in rehabilitation, 96

E

EMG (electromyographic) activity increase with PNF, 10
Etnyre, B.R., 12

F

Facilitated stretching. *See* PNF (proprioceptive neuromuscular facilitation)
Functional assessment for stretching. *See also* Joint evaluation for rehabilitation
  of adductors, 39
  of gastrocnemius, 34-35
  of hamstrings, 17
  of iliacus, 28-29
  of IT band, 44
  of piriformis, 48
  of psoas major, 28-29
  of quadriceps, 22
  of rotator cuff muscles, 55
  of soleus, 34-35
  of tensor fascia latae, 44
  of tibialis anterior, 25
  of triceps, 66
  of wrist muscles, 62

G

Garrett, W.E., 11
Gastrocnemius, 33-37
  diagram and description of, 33
  functional assessment of, 34-35
  partner stretches for, 36
  self-stretches for, 37
Gellhorn, Ernst, 9
Gesell, Arnold, 9
Golgi tendon organs (GTO), 4
Groin pulls, 39

H

Hamstrings, 16-20
  diagram and description of, 16
  functional assessment of, 17
  partner stretches for, 7, 8, 18, 20
  self-stretches for, 19
Heat for rehabilitation, 95
HR (hold-relax), 7
Hutton, R.S., 10, 11
Hypertension with PNF, 10-11

I

Iliacus, 27-32
  cautions for stretching, 29
  diagram and description of, 27
  functional assessment of, 28-29
  partner stretches for, 30-32
  self-stretches for, 31
Iliotibial band. *See* IT band
Inflammation, rehabilitation for, 94-95
Infraspinatus
  diagram and description of, 53
  partner stretches for, 57
  in rehabilitation, 96
Injuries. *See also* Rehabilitation
  groin pulls, 39

inflammation due to, 94-95
IT band pain syndrome, 44
less-than-maximal contractions for preventing, 14
risk of, from stretching, 6, 7, 39
scar tissue from, 95
Inverse stretch reflex, 4
Irradiation, law of, 4, 5
Isometric contractions
  in CRAC with single-muscle stretches, 14
  in CRAC with spiral-diagonal stretches, 79
  description of, 3
  less-than-maximal, for preventing injury, 14
  research on, 10, 11
  risks related to, 10, 11
Isotonic contractions, 3
IT band, 43-47
  cautions for stretching, 44
  diagram and description of, 43
  functional assessment of, 44
  partner stretches for, 45-47
IT band pain syndrome, 44

J

Joint evaluation for rehabilitation, 95. *See also* Functional assessment for stretching

K

Kabat, Herman, 2, 4, 7, 9, 11, 77
Kabat-Kaiser Institute (KKI), 2
Kaiser, Henry, 2
Knott, Margaret, 2, 77
Koslow, R., 10

L

Legs. *See* Lower extremity stretches, single-muscle; Lower extremity stretches, spiral-diagonal
Lower extremity stretches, single-muscle, 16-51
  for adductors, 38-42
  benefits of, 16
  CRAC techiques for, 14-15
  for gastrocnemius, 33-37
  for hamstrings, 16-20
  for iliacus, 27-32
  for IT band, 43-47
  for piriformis, 48-51
  for psoas major, 27-32
  for quadriceps, 21-24
  for soleus, 33-37
  for tensor fascia latae, 43-47
  for tibialis anterior, 25-26
Lower extremity stretches, spiral-diagonal, 82-84, 88-92
  D1 extension (toe-off), 82, 83-84, 88-89
  D1 flexion (soccer kick), 82, 90-91
  D2 extension (turnout), 82, 91-92
  D2 flexion (snowplow), 82
  techniques for, 82-84
Lucas, R.C., 10

M

Massage, stretches for reducing discomfort of, 13
Massage Training Institute, 14
Medeiros, J.M., 10
Mobilization for rehabilitation, 98
Modified PNF, development of, 2
Moore, M.A., 10, 11
Movement patterns, spiral-diagonal, 2, 77-82
Moyer, R.A., 11
Muscle contractions. *See also* Isometric contractions
  research on, 10
  types of, 3
Muscle spindle cells, function of, 3-4
Muscle strengthening for rehabilitation, 95, 98
Muscle types, in rehabilitation, 95-97
Myotatic stretch reflex, 3-4

N

Neurophysiological basis for PNF, 3-5, 11
NF techniques, development of, 2

O

Overuse tendinitis, stretches for preventing, 63

P

Pain
    IT band pain syndrome, 44
    muscle soreness, preventing, 15
    and psoas major, 29
    sciatic nerve pain, 49
    stretches for prevention/relief of, 49, 68
    stretching techniques with, 7
Paralysis, PNF for rehabilitation with, 2
Partner stretches (passive stretching)
    for adductors, 40-41
    for back extensors, 73-74
    description of, 6-7
    for gastrocnemius, 36
    for hamstrings, 7, 8, 18, 20
    for iliacus, 30-32
    for infraspinatus, 57
    for IT band, 45-47
    for pectoralis, 58
    for piriformis, 50
    for psoas major, 30-32
    for quadratus lumborum, 70-71
    for quadriceps, 23-24
    research on, 10, 11
    risks with, 6, 7, 10, 39 (see also Cautions)
    for rotator cuff muscles, 56-58
    for soleus, 36
    for subscapularis, 56
    techniques for, 14-15, 78-84
    for tensor fascia latae, 45-47
    for tibialis anterior, 26
    for triceps, 67
    for upper trapezius, 76
    for the wrist, 63-64
Passive stretching. See Partner stretches (passive stretching)
Pavlov, Ivan, 9
Pectoralis
    diagram and description of, 54
    partner stretches for, 58
    in rehabilitation, 95
Piriformis, 48-51
    cautions for stretching, 49
    diagram and description of, 48
    functional assessment of, 48
    partner stretches for, 50
    piriformis syndrome, 49
    self-stretches for, 51
PNF (proprioceptive neuromuscular facilitation). See also
        Benefits of PNF stretches; CR (contract-relax); CRAC
        (contract-relax, antagonist-contract); Partner
        stretches (passive stretching); Rehabilitation; Self-
        stretches; Single-muscle stretches; Spiral-diagonal
        stretches
    arguments against use of, 10-11
    definition of, 1
    future directions for, 3
    history of development of, 1-3, 9
    HR (hold-relax), 7
    modified PNF, 2
    neurophysiological basis for, 3-5, 11
    NF techniques, 2
    research on, 10-12
    research support for, 11-12
    risks with, 10-11, 39 (see also Cautions)
    Scientific Stretching for Sport (3-S technique), 2
    techniques, general description of, 7-8
Polio, PNF for rehabilitation, 2

Prentice, W.E., 11
Proprioceptive neuromuscular facilitation (PNF). See PNF
        (proprioceptive neuromuscular facilitation)
Psoas major, 27-32
    cautions for stretching, 29
    diagram and description of, 27
    functional assessment of, 28-29
    partner stretches for, 30-32
    self-stretches for, 31

Q

Quadratus lumborum
    diagram and description of, 69
    partner stretches for, 70-71
Quadriceps, 21-24
    diagram and description of, 21
    functional assessment of, 22
    partner stretches for, 23-24
    self-stretches for, 24
Quedenfeld, T.C., 11

R

Reciprocal innervtion, law of, 4, 5
Reflexes. See Stretch reflexes
Rehabilitation, 93-99
    components of, general, 93
    components of, specific, 97-99
    goals of, 94
    guidelines for, 94-95
    heat for, 95
    for inflammation, 94-95
    joint evaluation for, 95
    muscle strengthening for, 95, 98
    muscles types in, 95-97
    for polio, with paralysis, 2
    for scar tissue, 95
    specific PNF techniques for, listed, 94
    specific techniques for, described, 97-99
    theoretical case study of, 95-97
    typical session for, 97-99
    warm-up for, 97-98
Repetitive motion syndrome, stretches for preventing, 63
Risks. See also Cautions
    with ballistic stretching, 6
    with passive stretching, 6, 7, 10, 39
    with PNF, 10-11, 39
Rotator cuff muscles, 52-59
    diagram and description of, 52-54
    functional assessment of, 55
    infraspinatus stretch, 53, 57
    partner stretches for, 56-58
    pectoralis stretch, 54, 58
    self-stretches for, 59
    subscapularis stretch, 53, 56, 59

S

Sady, S.P., 11
Sapega, A.A., 11
Scar tissue, rehabilitation for, 95
Sciatic nerve pain, 49
Scientific Stretching for Sport (3-S technique), 2
Seaber, A.V., 11
Self-stretches
    for adductors, 42
    for gastrocnemius, 37
    for hamstrings, 19
    for iliacus, 31
    for piriformis, 51
    for psoas major, 31
    for quadriceps, 24
    for rotator cuff muscles, 59
    for soleus, 37
    for subscapularis, 59
    for tibialis anterior, 26
    for the triceps, 68
    for the wrist, 65

Sherrington, Charles, 2, 4, 9
Sherrington's laws, 4
Single-muscle stretches. *See also* Lower extremity
　　stretches, single-muscle; Torso stretches; Upper
　　extremity stretches, single-muscle
　　benefits of, 16
　　compared to spiral-diagonal stretches, 81, 84
　　CRAC techiques for, 14-15
　　preventing soreness due to, 15
　　purpose of, 13
Smidt, G.L., 10
Soderberg, G.L., 10
Soleus, 33-37
　　diagram and description of, 33
　　functional assessment of, 34-35
　　partner stretches for, 36
　　self-stretches for, 37
Soreness due to stretching, preventing, 15
Spindle cells, function of, 3-4
Spiral-diagonal stretches. *See also* Lower extremity
　　stretches, spiral-diagonal; Upper extremity stretches,
　　spiral-diagonal
　　compared to single-muscle stretches, 81, 84
　　movement patterns for, 2, 77-78
　　techniques for, 78-84
Sport-specific training for rehabilitation, 98-99
Stabilization muscles, in rehabilitation, 96-97
Static stretching
　　description of, 5-6
　　research on effectiveness of, 10, 11-12
Stretching. *See* Ballistic stretching; PNF (proprioceptive
　　neuromuscular facilitation); Static stretching
Stretching (Anderson), 5
Stretch reflexes
　　research on, 11
　　types of, 3-5
Subscapularis
　　diagram and description of, 53
　　partner stretches for, 56
　　in rehabilitation, 95
　　self-stretches for, 59
Successive induction, law of, 4
Surburg, P.R., 10

T

Tanigawa, M.C., 11
Taylor, D.C., 11
Tendinitis, stretches for preventing, 63
Tensor fascia latae, 43-47
　　cautions for stretching, 44
　　diagram and description of, 43
　　functional assessment of, 44
　　partner stretches for, 45-47

3-S technique (Scientific Stretching for Sport), 2
Tibialis anterior
　　diagram and description of, 25
　　functional assessment of, 25
　　partner stretches for, 26
　　self-stretches for, 26
Torso stretches, 68-76
　　for back extensors, 72-74
　　benefits of, 68
　　for quadratus lumborum, 69-71
　　for upper trapezius, 75-76
Trapezius, upper. *See* Upper trapezius
Triceps, 65-68
　　diagram and description of, 65
　　functional assessment of, 66
　　partner stretches for, 67
　　in rehabilitation, 95-96
　　self-stretches for, 68

U

Upper extremity stretches, single-muscle, 52-68
　　CRAC techiques for, 14-15
　　for infraspinatus, 53, 57
　　for pectoralis, 54, 58
　　for rotator-cuff muscles, 52-59
　　for subscapularis, 53, 56, 59
　　for triceps, 65-68
　　for the wrist, 60-65
Upper extremity stretches, spiral-diagonal, 79-81, 84-88
　　D1 extension (swimmer's stretch), 79-80, 84-85
　　D1 flexion (self-feeding), 79-80, 85-86
　　D2 extension (sheathing a sword), 80-81, 87-88
　　D2 flexion (drawing a sword), 80-81, 86-87
　　in rehabilitation, 95-96, 97
　　techniques for, 79-81
Upper trapezius
　　diagram and description of, 75
　　partner stretches for, 76

V

Valsalva maneuver, 11
Voss, Dorothy, 2, 77, 79

W

Warm-up for rehabilitation, 97-98
Wortman, M., 11
Wrist muscles, 60-65
　　benefits of stretching, 60
　　cautions for stretching, 63
　　diagram and description of, 60-61
　　functional assessment of, 62
　　partner stretches for, 63-64
　　self-stretches for, 65